✷
RITUAL

• MOON •

RITUAL

Daily Practices for
WELLNESS, BEAUTY
& BLISS

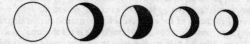

VASUDHA RAI

EBURY
PRESS
An imprint of Penguin Random House

EBURY PRESS

USA | Canada | UK | Ireland | Australia
New Zealand | India | South Africa | China

Ebury Press is part of the Penguin Random House group of companies
whose addresses can be found at global.penguinrandomhouse.com

Published by Penguin Random House India Pvt. Ltd
4th Floor, Capital Tower 1, MG Road,
Gurugram 122 002, Haryana, India

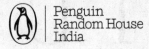

Penguin
Random House
India

First published in Ebury Press by Penguin Random House India 2022

Copyright © Vasudha Rai 2022

Illustrations by Parthika Immaneni

ISBN 9780143452935

Typeset in Adobe Garamond Pro by Manipal Technologies Limited, Manipal
Printed at Replika Press Pvt. Ltd, India

www.penguin.co.in

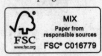

MIX
Paper from
responsible sources
FSC® C016779

For Rishaan, the Buddha in my life

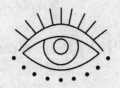

CONTENTS

PILLAR II: *Heal*

PILLAR III: *Rest*

ɔINTRODUCTION

An Ode to the Night

Come twilight, the dusk begins to deepen and before you know it, darkness falls like a comforting blanket on a scorching day. The inky night frames the Moon and stars previously hidden. The evening melts our resistance, making way for a sweeter surrender to the darkness. As the outer world draws to a close, activity slows down to make way for comfort. As weariness takes over, there's no reason to fight.

The passive, introspective energy of the Moon rules the depths of our mind. Sense organs have little use after nightfall. Release the need for control and submit to the placid moonlight. Introspect, reflect, and find pleasure so that mind, body, and spirit can begin to heal. Forget logic, sense, and reasoning, and learn to flow with the tide. Our dreams give us direction, illuminating what we can't see with our eyes.

The Moon—feminine and ever changing, at times voluptuously full and at others, blending into the night—

dances in its phases, symbolic of impermanence and the many faces of life. Its accompanying darkness is magical, always hiding something in plain sight.

The night can be melancholic, if you are lonesome. But fear not weary traveller, La Luna stands alone too. Sometimes she shines to her greatest potential sometimes, and hides herself at other times. Fill your inner world with magic. Stay still and peel back the layers one by one. The darkness makes the impossible come to life, like discovering roses in the desert or water inside the Sun.

The celestial bodies around you and the silence of the night. Don't be afraid of the Dark—it is the other half of Light. In the day we give ourselves to the world, but the nights are for receiving. The Darkness says: Calm down, ease up, and open yourself up to cosmic gifts.

Rest, renew, heal, and sleep deeply, like a baby. The morning will come quickly, so release the pressure and let yourself unravel. Become aware of your inner rhythm, your breath, heartbeat and vibrations. Slow down, find quiet, melt into the dark. The moonlight shines softly, as you glide among the stars.

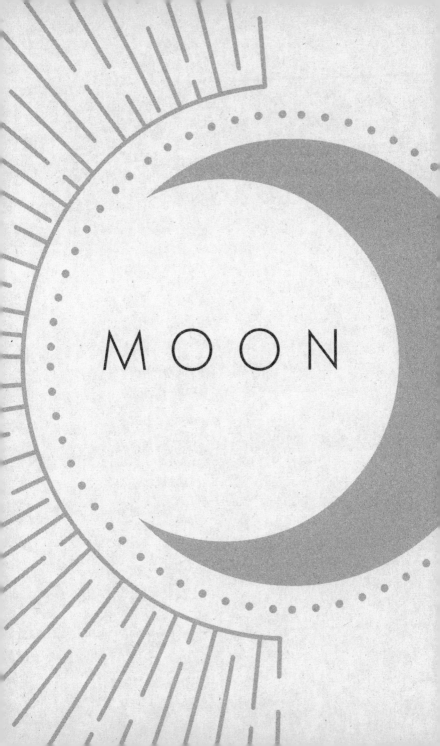

MOON

In the darkness the moon comes out, bringing with it immense potential for healing and rejuvenation. After the scorching sunshine of the day, the silvery mist of the night acts like a soothing balm for tired souls. Unlike the sun, a symbol of predictability, the moon changes on a daily basis, waxing and waning with its gentle movements. In a physical sense, we can only see just one side of our celestial neighbour. Its dark side, which faces away from earth, is always out of view. It's constantly changing shape—from crescent to full—which makes the moon a source of mystery to humans. Whether it's magic or medicine, sexuality or fertility, lunar folklore is popular across all cultures.

The Vedas considered the moon to be the vessel for the mysterious soma, a drink that made the gods invincible. We still haven't found the exact source of soma, which is something to think about, especially since other Vedic plants such as hemp and barley are found even today. Lunar deities are both male and female, whether it's Chandra in the Vedas or Ix Chel, the Mayan moon goddess of love, fertility and medicine. In Buddhism, the full moon is a symbol of enlightenment, its various phases depicting the ever-changing nature of life. In Chinese mythology, Goddess Chang'e or Chang-o stole the elixir of immortality. When she drank it, she became so light that she floated up to the moon. Legend has it that she lives there even today with only a rabbit for company.

The moon has also given us direction since the beginning of civilization. In Arabia, tradesmen travelled in the desert during the night using the position of the moon and stars as a reference. Even today, the moon is of great significance in Islam, with the crescent shape representing progress and the five-pointed star, light and knowledge. In the days of the lunar calendar, which is eleven days shorter than the current solar calendar, it was used to measure time and seasonality. The Mayans and Chinese used the lunar calendar for agricultural purposes. Even today, the positions of the moon are used to set dates for festivals and holidays—whether its Holi and Diwali in India or the Chinese New Year between January and February every year.

The moon is a celestial body that frightens and inspires us in equal measure. There isn't any doubt that we have a natural affinity for its cycles. Menstruation cycles in women are every twenty-eight days, which is the exact number of days as the lunar cycle. Unlike the earth, which spins on its axis every 24 hours, the moon takes twenty-seven and a half days for every rotation.

Marine life, in fact, has finely tuned moon clocks. The light-sensitive neutrons of corals absorb the energy of the moonlight and on a full-moon night, go into a mating frenzy. Some species of fish and crabs gestate during certain lunar phases, while plankton rise up from the seabed to feed once it gets dark. The moon is so powerful that it generates a gravitational pull we know as the tidal force that causes a bulge in the oceans that face towards it.

The moon's ability to heal and nourish may not be directly proven by scientific studies, but night-time activities of rest and sleep are the best nourishers known to man. We are attuned on every level—mind, body and emotion—to tap into this frequency of the night. The moment it gets dark, our bodies begin to produce melatonin, the sleep hormone, getting us ready for rest and recovery. Tuning ourselves to relax after dark is the best health supplement. Tuning your sleep and wake cycles with the natural circadian rhythms of sunrise and unwinding after sunset is the best medicine for chronic ailments. Every species has its own biological clock— some stay awake according to the solar cycles while others are wakeful during lunar hours.

Humans in general stay awake during the day and rest at night. But perhaps this is the hardest change to make, especially since there are two types of humans—the early birds and the night owls. I don't believe in forcing the body to do something that doesn't come naturally. So, if you're more awake during the night, it's essential to get your 8 hours of sleep, even if it's later at night or day. Of course, use the sun and the moon rituals interchangeably, depending on the need instead of tangible divisions of day and night. If you need nourishment, healing or rest during the day, the remedies presented in this part will help you get in touch with your yin/moon side.

Still, both science and tradition are on the side of the early risers. Following the natural rhythms of sunrise and sunset have positive results on health. This includes metabolism, weight loss, blood pressure, heart health and hormones. While light acts as a stimulus for activity, darkness encourages sleep. In the last couple of decades, a majority of the population in the world has acquired at least one device that keeps us up at night. The continuous scrolling is anxiety-inducing and the light from your device inhibits melatonin production, thereby postponing sleep.

If you've twisted and turned late at night with forbidden thoughts eroding your peace of mind, you're not alone. Scientists have found that going to bed later increases negative thoughts, while getting a good night's rest helps you solve problems better. Sleep strengthens the immune system, makes you healthier and even makes you more satisfied with life. Just like work is the big project in the day, sleep is the assignment of the night. Every activity after sunset must therefore lead to the ultimate night-time goal of rest.

A very wise man once told me that we must plan our sleep just like we prepare for a holiday. This means that evening activities must be geared towards rest, as opposed to acting as stimulants, which keep us up all night. The cooling energy of the moon must be utilized correctly in order to harmonize or cycles of activity and leisure. Like yin to the yang of the day, the softness of night must be harnessed to its maximum potential, whether to sleep, love or heal.

To match our energies with the moon's placidity and calmness, activities must be divided into the following, not only as a method to reach peak health but also as a reward for a hard day's work.

1) Nurture—to nourish mind, body, spirit
2) Heal—to recover from emotional and physical assaults
3) Rest—to prepare for sleep

Think of these as the three pillars of the moon—one leads to the other. Whether it's the food you eat, the beverages you drink, exercise or spiritual practices, the focus must be turned inwards as opposed to the outward direction of the day.

From 4 p.m. begins the cycle of night, which in a way mirrors the morning. Just like 4–6 a.m. is ideal for meditation in the morning, 4–6 p.m. is also ideal for a journey inwards. Ayurveda suggests that the lightweight qualities of vata, dominated by the elements of air and space, are diffused through the atmosphere during this. The environment is quiet and environment provides clarity. You also find that late afternoon is the ideal time for a break. Whether it's a short spell of sound healing, guided meditation or mantra practice, a small break during this time pulls you through till the evening.

From 6–10 p.m. is kapha time, with its grounding earth energy, which is perfect for healing, the second pillar of the moon. This period is ideal to unwind with a walk, restorative yoga or self-massage. Since night-time is also when our skin naturally regenerates, it is also the best time to beautify and heal the skin with oils, massages, *ubtans* and masks.

After 10 p.m. begins pitta time, governed by fire, which explains why you sometimes get a second wind when it's time for bed. I find that sleep is the soundest when you switch the lights off before the pitta period begins. Personally, I find it impossible to sleep this early, but for most part I turn in by 11 p.m. But before that I like to spend some time with either a kriya, beverage, breathing exercises or journaling.

The energy of the moon is introspective, but must be driven by gratitude. Fortunately or unfortunately, we all know that no matter how bad things may be, they can always be worse. Just like the spirit of hope must be cultivated for an active day, being thankful for something that went right (because something always does) brings peace and rest in the night.

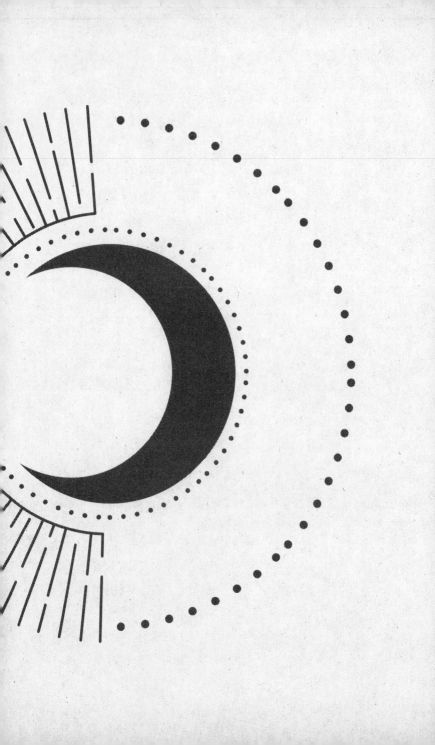

PILLAR I

∗

Nurture

'Touch comes before sight, before speech. It is the first language and the last, and it always tells the truth.'

—Margaret Atwood, *The Blind Assassin*

When someone asks me to define wellness, I always say if you were your own child, how would you treat yourself? Self-care is mothering yourself, a treat at the end of a working day or cosseting on a off. It's a small reward for surviving in this world, it heals and holds you together. We can nurture ourselves in many different ways. Food is the obvious choice. But in order to enjoy this care, every sense organ must be indulged—whether it's the sense of smell, sound, or the healing power of touch.

In the modern world, where everything is divided into black and white, it's easy to forget that consumption happens via all our senses. Everything gets absorbed by the mind and affects the body, be it food, visuals, sounds, touch and smell that have the potential to build us up or break us down. If you look at consumption as a full sensorial experience, it's easy to see that just following a prescriptive lifestyle isn't key to health and happiness. You could eat all the 'toxins' in the world and still feel great only because you're perhaps in a good place in life or a healthy relationship, free from stress and worry. The positive effects of wellness reflect in better physical health, but just like disease, healing begins in the mind, with the inputs we receive from our senses.

Take the simple act of eating a meal. You can conjure the sight and smell of food only in your mind and it will your make your mouth water. Taste, fragrance, texture and sound all make meals a 360-degree affair. This perception goes beyond food because all our senses have the potential to excavate buried treasures. A whiff of perfume revives a long-dead memory; a song can take you decades into the past. Everything we consume via our senses gets programmed into our consciousness. Therefore, it is essential to choose how we want to be stimulated, especially today, when unrestricted stimuli invade us unchosen and unannounced via our tablets and smartphones.

As we age, our sense organs become weaker, which increases the importance of nurturing. Our lifestyles have also become such that we invariably burn the candle at both ends, working in the present and worrying about what will happen next. It has been found that the act of worrying about the future leads to significant cognitive decline and reduced memory function. Additionally, emotional stress may increase the risk of heart attack as much as smoking or high blood pressure. Even a longer work week could lead to higher blood pressure; long-term exposure to traffic noise may increase the risk of heart disease.

The life we've built is has disturbed us to the point of ill health. The work hard/play harder mantra may have been relevant decades ago, but today it's fairly obsolete as we have collectively realized the value of work/life balance. But though we understand the importance of self-care in theory, we rarely put it into practice. Even today, every other activity takes precedence over taking care of ourselves. We ignore pain, fatigue, trauma to meet deadlines and finish projects. My coach in the gym says that people word hard to make money till their forties and then spend the latter part of their lives spending that money to regain their health. Hard work is certainly essential, but so is rest and recovery. Even 10 minutes a day can help revive and soothe frayed nerves.

Self-care doesn't have to be a grand affair—just placing a warm palm on a painful spot is taking care of yourself. Putting your phone away and listening to your favourite song, eating a delicious meal without distraction, holding the hand of someone you love—all help in small ways to make you feel better. Any time you forget the outside world, directing your energy and attention towards the present moment is healing and restorative. We're often so stimulated with information excess that we forget to hear our innermost signals. But to listen, you have to connect, and make time to receive. There are many ways to make this connection, but the most important element is stillness.

Massage, in particular, is the perfect example of a nurturing ritual, which helps us connect with mind and body. It's looked upon as an occasional treat but traditional sciences such as Ayurveda have always stressed on the importance on making it daily self-practice. Not does massage help with releasing stress and pain in the physical body, it helps reduce soothe the mind.

The Sanskrit word for oil is *sneha*, which also means love. Therefore, the act of oil massage is traditionally seen as an act of love, ideally performed with attention and complete connection to the body. If you look at it from a scientific lens, there's enough evidence to prove that it works for a range of conditions. From reducing pain and anxiety in cancer and fibromyalgia patients, to weight gain in premature babies and improved sleep in menopausal women, massage isn't just a luxury but a necessity in modern-day living.

Self-care for me is synonymous with self-love because you make time to listen to your body's signals and prioritize its needs. Whether it's the application of a face mask, rubbing down the body with a body brush or shampooing your hair, beautification can lead to bliss. When it becomes a regular part of your daily routine, it becomes a joyous activity to look forward to every single day. At a subconscious level, it has been found that just anticipating positive events provides exponential benefits for mental and emotional health.

While self-care covers everything from diet and exercise to other kriyas, this section will focus solely upon beauty rituals and their feel-good potential. Beauty rituals are nourishing for many different reasons—they can help you relax, stay connected to the moment or energize you for the day. They can uplift your mood and soothe frazzled nerves. But most importantly, in this world where nothing can be predicted, they provide you a safe haven to come back to, over and over again.

1

MASSAGE

Human beings are instinctively drawn to massage—when we hurt ourselves, we naturally reach out to rub the pain away. When we're heartbroken, nothing feels as comforting as touch. In Ayurveda it is believed that the masseuse gives her positive energy and absorbs the negative energy in return from the patient. Whether we're tired, anxious or uneasy, the long, deep strokes of massage lull the mind into tranquillity. It nurtures the mind and nourishes the skin. Because it increases circulation, it brings fresh, oxygenated blood right under the surface, to directly feed the skin. Massage unravels tight muscles, helps lubricate the joints and reduces mental stress. It is backed by scientific data, where it has been shown to clinically reduce levels of pain.

The Gate Control Theory proposes that the body's sensations are carried up the spine by neurological fibres to the brain. Smaller fibres carry stimulation like pain, while larger ones carry harmless sensations like rubbing or scratching. In theory, it is believed that the large fibre activity can close off the channel or 'gate' for small fibre sensations to reach the brain. This means that by rubbing or kneading an injury, you have sent some stimulation that can block the sensation of pain, thereby reducing its perception. Though the theory is still debated, it provides an explanation for the comforting aspect of massage, especially as far as pain relief is concerned.

One way or another, I find that massaging even a small part of my body results in a sense of well-being. Whether it's feeling lighter after a foot rub or more grounded after a using facial tool, massage for me is a direct connection to my body and a way for me to shower it with love. Naturally, the biggest impediment to massage is making it a part of your daily ritual, especially since we prefer activities with tangible benefits, such as work or workouts. But daily massages also provide tangible benefits, whether it's elevating skin quality to nourishing the joints and connective tissue, reducing pain and toning muscles. On the worst days, it is tempting to give it up altogether, but massage helps settle my mind and ease my body.

For me, the biggest advantage is that it lulls the mind into a state of bliss. It removes mental cobwebs so that good ideas can float to the surface. It's a little bit like meditation, actually. When I'm deep into massage, an idea appears from the recesses of my mind, just like it does while I'm meditating. Especially when I'm facing a mental block, stepping away from the task and doing something meditative helps untangle confused thoughts. Massage has a way of ironing out the kinks, giving clarity of thought at the very least and a completely disconnected, empty mind at its best.

Face Massage

In terms of beautification, massage helps tone and sculpt the face if it is done with the right technique. The friction causes circulation, which means you're oxygenating and feeding the skin with nutrients. It helps relieve muscular tension, which is also a cause of sagging in the face. Small studies have shown that daily massage with a device increases the level of proteins in the skin, thereby giving an appearance of tightness. It also helps reduce the appearance of raised scars, especially in burn rehabilitation. It has also been found that massage causes morphological changes, including tightening and lifting of the tissue at the jaw and thickening of the nasal ring and lift on the lower cheeks.

The friction created by massage breaks down adhesions. Friction massages are part of sports remedies used to mobilize tissue in the ligaments, tendons and muscles, and prevent scars from forming. This mobilization affects the lymphatic system too. Precise strokes move fluid that surrounds the cells towards the lymph nodes to be purified. Therefore, it is essential to get acquainted with the right techniques to tone the facial structure and create a bespoke massage sequence for oneself.

There is no doubt that daily massage boosts radiance, enhances the bone structure and reduces the appearance of lines and wrinkles. The only contraindication would be massage on an oily, acne prone complexion, as over-stimulating the skin could lead to more breakouts. But as we grow older, it does have its advantages for beautification. For me, it's a ritual that signals the beginning or the end of the day. When I do it in the morning, it helps me consolidate my thoughts about work. At the end of the day, it signals the end of screen time.

The Basic Face Tone

If you're familiar with the methodology of massages, you'll find that in the face, there is a basic set of movements that work along the natural musculature and the presence of the lymph nodes. Interestingly, unlike blood that circulates all over the body, the lymph moves in an outward direction. It travels via the main clavicular vein that runs down the side of the ears to the shoulder blades and then out the shoulders. Most of the nodes are situated in the hollows of the face (under the eyes, sides of the nose and mouth, around the ears and jaw). Therefore, most massages focus on movements that go from the centre of the face towards the sides and then down the master drain behind the ears. These movements help mobilize the interstitial fluid that surround the cells, towards the nodes to be purified.

If you look at the muscular structure of the face, you'll find that most muscles originate from the periphery and insert in the middle of the face. Therefore, by massaging them in outward movements, we are reinforcing and strengthening the 'roots' of these muscles. Long, smooth, firm strokes also help massage the neck and jaw area that is overused because of emotional and physical stress. In my practice, I've noticed that massage has helped smooth wrinkles, define contours and increase the tightness and glow of my face.

Kapala Randhra Dhauti

This is a technique which has been popularized by the Gherand Samhita, a Sanskrit text and one of the most comprehensive treatises in yoga. Literally translated, it means clearing the cavities of the head. Though this isn't mentioned in ancient Ayurvedic texts, it has been briefly referred to in the Yogic Shatkriyas.

If done correctly, it removes the kapha dosha (responsible for nasal congestion) from the upper part of the body.

1. Create a 'V' shape with your middle and forefingers to rub the area in front and behind your ears.
2. Place your thumbs on the temples and use all four fingers to horizontally massage the forehead from one end to the other, alternating each hand.

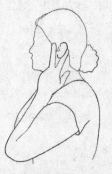

Step 1

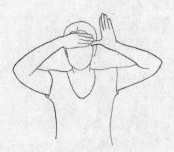

Step 2a

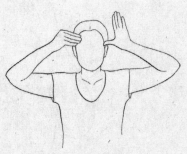

Step 2b

3. Use your middle and ring fingers to massage the eye. Start from the inner corner of the under the eye to the outer corners and then up towards the temples, above the brow towards the centre.

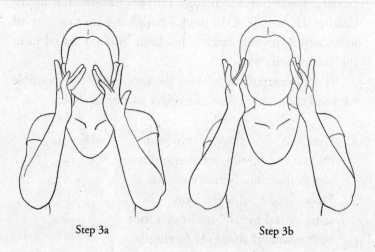

Step 3a   Step 3b

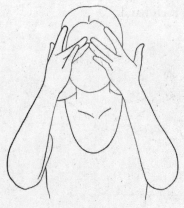

Step 3c

4. Sweep your entire palm, pressing down from the sides of the nose and lips, upwards towards the temples.

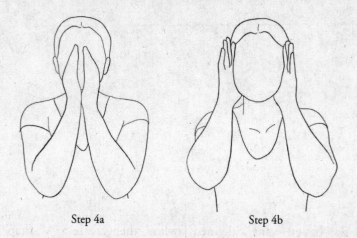

Step 4a   Step 4b

5. Create a 'V' shape with your fingers by placing one finger over and under the lips horizontally. Sweep from the lips upwards closing the V when you reach the temples, alternating the hands.

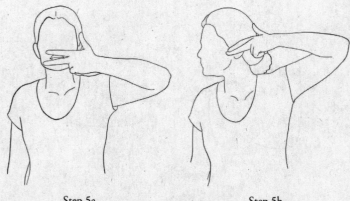

Step 5a   Step 5b

15

6. Massage the neck in upward strokes.

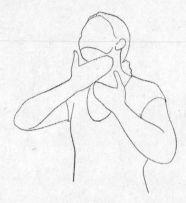

Step 6

7. If you want a defined jawline, then create a 'V' shape with your fingers, and massage from the chin towards the temple, keeping one finger on the jawline and the other one under. Or keep the thumb under the jaw and the rest of the fingers above.

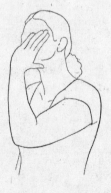 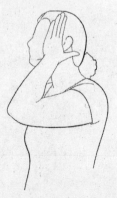

Step 7a   Step 7b

Head Massage

The brain is the most overworked part of the body, averaging (yogis say) about 60,000 thoughts in a day. It's no surprise then that the repeated drumming of a head massage feels thoughts being demolished in the brain. A 15-minute scalp rub reduces level of stress hormones and significantly decreases blood pressure. The Indian head massage in particular increases parasympathetic nerve activity (the rest and relax mode of the body), relieves anxiety and refreshes the mind. The kneading and rubbing movements of a massage eases tight muscles around the neck and shoulders. Since the scalp is located at the top of the body, the increased circulation may also lead to healthier hair follicles. Though it is a minuscule study, there is some evidence to show that a daily 4-minute massage increases hair thickness. This massage can be done with and without hair oil.

Head massage in traditional systems is used to both calm the mind and improve hair health. In Ayurveda, the head is considered to be the root of the body, while the limbs are branches. Apt, since we now know that all diseases begin in the mind. Our head is also the location of the hypothalamus and pituitary gland. Together, they're considered to be the control centre for the endocrine system, producing several important hormones such as FSH, TSH, prolactin, oxytocin and growth hormones, to name a few. Of course, the head is the root of our internal heaven or hell. It's the origination of thought, the creation of an inner world.

The skull also holds several important *marma* points, which are healing energy points that work as doorways into the body and consciousness when stimulated. The head, most notably, has the *adhipati*, located eight fingers from the brows in the centre of the skull, over which hovers the crown chakra. Adhipati, when translated, means king, therefore it is considered to be the master of all marma points in the body, increasing their performance and efficiency.

Along with stimulating the adhipati, head massage also stimulates several other important marma points. These include the *simantaka* point, twelve fingers from the brows, and *krikatika*, that is two points on either side of the cervical spine, where the skull joins the head. Then there are two *vidhuram* points in the depression behind the earlobes and the *shankha*, which is the depression on the temples, which is also rubbed and stimulated in Indian head massage.

Typically, most marma points are in the hollows of the body. It is believed that stimulating these points during a massage calms an overactive mind, enhances sleep quality, improves vision, relaxes the muscles and rejuvenates the entire nervous system.

How to Heat Oil for Massage

Warming the oil, whether it's for hair, body or navel massage, is highly recommended as the heat helps it penetrate deeper. Never apply direct heat to the oil as it can disturb its composition. Warm it indirectly by immersing the required amount of oil in a bowl and immerse it in a larger bowl of hot water. Or just place the bottle straight into the bowl of hot water.

The Basic Scalp Massage

1. Oil massage must be done on a clean scalp. Massaging a dirty scalp will make it even dirtier and prone to infections.

2. Choose an oil suited to your personal ayurvedic dosha and season. If you are vata-dominant, characterized by a slight build, dry skin and a running mind, choose warming oils like castor and sesame. If you're pitta-dominant, with reddish skin, medium build and a tendency towards anger, select a cooling oil such as coconut. If you're ruled by kapha, characterized by a full build, glossy skin and calm mind, choose a hot oil such as mustard. In terms of season, oils such as coconut are suited to summer, whereas the usage of mustard oil must be limited to winter. You can warm the oil or keep it at room temperature depending on the season and your own personal *prakriti*.

3. If you're comfortable with applying oil to your forehead, begin by rubbing the oil in circular motions at the third eye, going along the centre line towards the second marma point of the adhipati (eight-finger widths from the brows) and simantaka (twelve-finger width from the brows).

4. The oil must be poured first in the centre parting to stimulate the main marma points and then worked outwards towards the temples, earlobes and the nape of the neck.

5. Keep a medium pressure to prevent over-stimulating the scalp. The idea is to gently relax the mind, therefore slow, deep, circular movements work best.

6. Make sure you gently rub all the main marmas, not just in the centre parting but also behind the earlobes, next to the cervical spine and around the temples.

7. Keep the oil on for 30 minutes at least. If you're using a medicated oil prescribed by your ayurvedic doctor, then keeping it for longer will provide more benefits.

8. Head massage is not advised for those with infections of the scalp such as psoriasis, eczema, fungal infections or dermatitis.

How to Wash Off Hair Oil

Always dilute the shampoo with a little bit of water. By doing so, you activate the foam and thin it out so it goes to every part of the scalp. When I dilute the shampoo, I only need to wash my hair once to clean it well.

Four-Ingredient Hair Oil

Ingredients:
1 cup aloe pulp
1 cup curry leaves
1 and a 1/2 cup fresh amla paste
1 cup coconut oil

Note: If you want multiple oils, then mix half a cup each of coconut and sesame oils with a quarter cup of castor oil. You can also add a cup of fresh paste of neem leaves for their anti-bacterial properties.

Method:

Heat all the ingredients in an iron wok on a low flame till the water evaporates. You know that all the moisture has evaporated once bubbles stop forming in this infusion. Take care not to overheat.

Know Your Oil

Coconut: Cooling, promotes hair growth, enhances thickness. Must be avoided by those prone to fungal infections and dandruff as it can feed the microbes.

Almond: Conditions the hair shaft, strengthens the follicles, improves scalp health and is cooling in nature.

Castor: Helps increase hair density and delays greying by removing excess heat in the scalp. Its dense viscosity means that it must be used in combination with another, lighter oil.

Black sesame: Enhances hair growth, relieves headaches, delays greying and combats dryness.

Moringa: Anti-inflammatory and moisturizing, therefore works on flakiness caused by excessive dryness on the scalp.

Mustard: Warming, therefore best suited to winter. Its warming quality also deepens the colour of henna on the hair. Apply it the day after henna application.

> Desi ghee: Builds hair strength, deeply conditions damaged hair, cools the scalp and makes strands incredibly soft.

Full Body Massage

While most massages focus on the muscles of the body, opening up tight knots and activating pressure points, in abhayanga, the oil and its formulation are of equal importance. Today we believe that the body absorbs ingredients through our skin, which explains the renewed interest in 'clean' beauty products. However, ayurvedic physicians understood this thousands of years ago, which is why they used oil not only as a skincare product but also as medicine. There are oils to relax, energize, beautify and detoxify the body, to name a few. In panchakarma, the great ayurvedic detox, oils are used to soften the tissue from the outside with massage and the inside as well with oil enemas and medicated ghee decoctions. The body absorbs this internal and external oleation believed to loosen toxins accumulated within.

Because of this reason, massage isn't a beauty or wellness treatment but also improves health and longevity. Even though you cannot do the full panchakarma at home, you can incorporate the key element of abhayanga into your routine. From an ayurvedic perspective, oil massages help calm an overactive vata, which is one the three main doshas. Vata rules movement, therefore without it there will be no circulation or elimination. Conversely, when vata is malfunctioning, it can also lead to conditions such as endometriosis by shifting the tissue. Vata imbalances are apparent in an overactive mind, problems with elimination and dry skin.

From a traditional point of view, oiling the body balances vata, thereby calming the mind, adding suppleness to skin and restoring bodily functions. If you look at oil massage from a scientific lens, you'll find that it has been shown to improve growth and sleep in infants. Almond oil, particularly, helps promote lactation, while clove oil helps reduce post-natal pain in mothers.

Traditionally, an oil massage is done before a bath and not afterwards. Since it is believed that the oils help loosen toxins, bathing after massage helps eliminate them. Typically, during a bath, some dry flour (like besan, powdered mung or jowar atta) is used to rub off the last remnants of greasiness and also exfoliate the skin. Understandably, in these times, this ritual is rather elaborate and time-consuming. So if you can't practise this on the daily, keep the self-abhayanga to a once-a-week treat, or rub the oil vigorously into your skin every day either before or after a bath.

Self Abhayanga

● Warm up a small bottle of oil by placing it in a bowl of hot water. Ayurveda doesn't recommend heating the oil directly as it can damage the delicate composition of phytonutrients. Half a cup of oil should be enough for the whole body—from the head to the toes—though you may need extra for the scalp depending on the length of your hair.

- The literal translation of abhayanga is 'to rub against' the limbs. Start at the feet and rub the oil vigorously into the skin so the friction produces heat, which in turn will help the oil get 'digested' by the body. Pay attention to every inch of your body including your toes and the space between the toes.

- Move up the legs in long, firm strokes, towards the pelvis and the hips. Remember the marma or pressure points lie within the hollows of the bone structure, so rub the oil into every nook and crevice, such as the joints of the body.

- Massage your stomach in circular motions along the direction of the intestines. So upwards towards the right, circle to the other side and downwards from the left, circling again towards the right.

- Rub the breasts in circular motions. Also rub the oil into the insides of the arms, armpits and shoulders.

- Massage the oil into your back, taking extra time on the lower back as we tend to hold a lot of stress in the lumbar area.

- Spend more time on the joints of the body. Massage the knees and elbows in circular motions to keep them supple.

- Coconut and olive oils are cooling, and therefore best for the warmer months or for those who have excess heat in the body. Sesame and almond are warming and are better for cooler months and better for those who feel excessively cold.

Foot Massage

If you look at the diagrams of the foot in TCM or Ayurveda, you'll find them to be very similar—the lower organs on the lower areas of the foot and the upper organs on the toes. The brain, eyes and ears are on the toes; the spleen, kidneys and intestines in the middle of the feet; the spine running along the arch of the foot and the sciatica on the heel. Traditional sciences believe that all organs are connected to the feet and perhaps there may be an element of truth in this. Each foot has a quarter of the bones in the body and around 7,000 nerve endings each. They also have a network of over 100 ligaments, muscles and tendons that connect them to the rest of the body. Therefore, any problem with the feet can spread to the spine and the rest of the body.

Though they're the most utilized organ, they're also the most ignored part of the body. On a good day, we will apply a quick swipe of moisturizer or get a pedicure. But they're never cared for like the head, scalp or face. In traditional sciences, feet have an exalted position. Washing them before bed is essential as it releases excess heat, cools the entire body and also removes the negative energies of the day. In fact, the ancient scriptures claim that washing the feet before bed gives better sleep and sweeter dreams.

Incidentally, the practice of *padabhayanga* (foot massage) is recommended in Ayurveda for eye strain. The feet and eyes are the two opposite poles in the body that are connected with nerves. Traditionally, the ayurvedic foot massage is believed to have a direct impact on eye health. It is believed that the act of massaging the feet improves the circulation of the eyes as two main nerves travel from the left and right foot to the left and right eye. There is small amount of evidence to show that this could actually work. In a small sample group, it was found that regularly practising padabhayanga with sesame seed oil indeed reduced strain in the eyes.

It has also been found that massaging the soles reduces the alpha and beta activity of the brain and induces sleep—a delta and theta wave activity. Additionally, there is some evidence to show that padabhayanga increases the levels of serotonin in the blood, meaning that its benefits go beyond just eye health.

Step-by-Step Foot Massage

- Start by warming sesame seed oil by immersing the container in hot water. If your eyes burn, you could also warm cow's ghee for its cooling properties. The oil/ghee must be at around 40 degrees Celsius, which is slightly warmer than body temperature.
- Massage should be done in anulom or upward direction. You could massage your feet with your hands or use an upside-down *kansa* bowl. Using kansa helps draw out excess heat and impurities from the body, resulting in dark grey soot that can be wiped away easily with a towel.
- The heel and bottom part of the feet represent the lower part of the body, the middle part of the feet is for the organs in the centre of the trunk, while the toes and pads of the feet represent the topmost organs such as the lungs and eyes.
- Perform the massage on clean feet. Apply the oil liberally not just on the soles but also on the top of the feet, the ankles and between each toe.

- Start by massaging the top of your foot from the ankle joint to the toes. Then do the same action on the sole from the ankle to the heels to the toes, making sure you massage the Achilles tendon.
- Make a fist and massage the soles with the knuckles, ensuring you get every part of the foot including the arch, the space under and between each toe.
- Go back to the top of the foot and rub the thumb from the ankle till the big toe and repeat the movement for each toe.
- Finish by rubbing, punching and pulling each toe between your fingers.
- As the last step, you could also soak your feet in warm, salted water for complete relaxation, but this is optional.

Note: You can practice padabhayanga at any time though I prefer to do it before bed. Avoid it right after a meal. Do it either an hour before or 2 hours after a meal.

SOS Knee Massage

If you have achy knees, massage them with warm sesame oil for 15 minutes on each knee. If you're older than thirty, do this once a week; if you're older than forty, do this twice a week; if you're older than fifty, do it every alternate day; and those over sixty should do it every day for supple joints.

2

UBTAN

I love the romance and versatility of an ubtan. It is a natural powder made with flowers, herbs and lentils, which changes function depending on the binding agent to create a hybrid mask/exfoliator. It can be mixed with milk, rosewater, honey, aloe vera or a fruit such as overripe papaya, which also bring their own qualities to the ubtan paste.

In older times, a paste of herbs and lentils was used on the daily. Though some people still follow this practice, it has become laborious for those with a busy lifestyle. Whether it is to reduce the fuzz around the face, exfoliate dead cells or add glow, the magic of an ubtan is that it is inexpensive and effective.

The Making of an Ubtan

Legumes and grains form the base of an ubtan. They have a gummy texture that binds with the liquid onto light, fuzzy hair and dead skin to remove them from the skin. This is what differentiates a traditional ubtan from a clay mask—

clays have a tendency to fall off the skin when rubbed, whereas something like besan becomes sticky.

Several herbs are added to this base of lentils and grain, the most common being turmeric (to disinfect, heal and brighten) and sandalwood (to soothe and clarify). In fact, the most common recipe for an ubtan is besan with a bit of turmeric and sandalwood, which has been found to have potent free radical-scavenging capacity, protecting and healing the skin. The beauty of the ubtan, however, is that you can make your own recipe according to the season and your skin type. So, if your skin is dry, you can use almond meal as a base; if you're sensitive, use a combination of milk and colloidal oatmeal; and those with oily complexions can enjoy herbs mixed with aloe vera gel.

Though there many traditional formulations, the best recipes are made by combining modern and old-world ingredients. For instance, I like to add raw cacao powder to an ubtan because it gives it a creaminess that is very beneficial in winter. When my skin breaks out, I like to stir in a bit of spirulina powder and apple cider vinegar to reduce redness and shrink acne. Part of what makes ubtan a ritual is the fact that we mix the proportions with our own hands, choosing what is good for us and putting in our own energy. It's like massage, in that sense, because there is human touch involved.

You could make it as basic or complicated as you wish, though I like to keep it simple, only because it's easier to observe what works and what doesn't. Keep it to four ingredients at a time: one that like an 'active', another to complement the main ingredient and boost its healing powers, plus a supporting ingredient either as a soothing agent or to boost the powers of the main active ingredient. The last ingredient is a binder, which could be either water, milk, yoghurt, honey, aloe or fruit pulp.

To understand this, let's take the example of one of my favourite ubtan recipes made with equal parts kasturi manjal (wild turmeric), sandalwood powder (either red or white) and orange peel or mulethi powder. The main active ingredient in this is the kasturi manjal, which helps brighten the skin and reduce pigmentation. I add cooling sandalwood to this because the turmeric is heating in nature and may cause a burning sensation. The last ingredient is either orange peel or mulethi because both also work to brighten the skin. However, since mulethi is a sweet herb it is gentler on the skin than orange peel. If I want to make this mask even more gentle, I will add rose petal powder, which is also very cooling. To bind, I choose honey instead of water because I want the mask to stick to my skin longer. I prefer not to use lentil powders in this because I sometimes use AHAs on my face and don't want the extra exfoliation. If I were to use it on my body, I would add lentil powder to it.

If you're making an ubtan for beauty, be creative and don't hesitate to modernize the recipe. That's not to say that traditional recipes aren't relevant. In fact, in several instances tradition is the way to go, especially when it comes to utilizing the knowledge for mind-body benefits.

Brightening Ubtan

1 tsp kasturi manjal powder
1 tsp red sandalwood powder
1 tsp orange peel/mulethi powder
Raw honey/milk/yoghurt to bind
A dash of rose water to loosen the paste

Method:

- Mix all the ingredients to a smooth paste
- Apply over face and neck
- Leave on for 15 minutes to an hour
- Wash off or use as a gentle exfoliator, but gently rub it off in circular motions

Calming Ubtan

1 tsp rose petal powder
1 tsp white sandalwood
1 tsp *jatamansi* powder
1 tbsp colloidal oats
1 tbsp aloe vera gel
Milk/yoghurt to bind
(If you're vegan use coconut milk)

Method:

- Mix the ingredients
- Pat on to the skin
- Wash off without rubbing the skin after 15 to 30 minutes

Moisturizing Ubtan

I tbsp raw cacao
Half an overripe banana
1/4 tsp gotu kola powder (skip this if your skin is sensitive)
A few drops of almond oil
Honey/milk/aloe vera gel, or all, to bind

Method:

- Mix the ingredients (you could also add a few drops of your favourite face oil)
- Smooth over face and neck
- Rub gently or wash off after 30 minutes to an hour

Full Body Exfoliation

Ayurveda has its own variation called the *udvarthana*, that is prescribed by ayurvedic doctors for a range of conditions. The practice involves rubbing the body with dry herbs to stimulate and heat it. The practice is commonly used in panchakarma for conditions such as diabetes and obesity. It can be done as a second step after body massage as the oil acts as a lubricant over the skin, which makes the exfoliation less abrasive. In people who have very dry skin, the powder is mixed with a little bit of oil which is hot in potency, such as mustard or sesame. The ultimate aim of udvarthana is to break down the fatty tissue, activate lymphatic drainage and increase circulation. By creating friction on the skin, it is said to balance the doshas, especially kapha (characterized by a heavier build) and vata (dry skin, frail build).

The powders used for this are hot in potency to help stimulate the skin, thereby helping liquify and mobilize stagnant adipose tissue. To ensure efficacy, the correct method must be followed. The best time to do this is in the morning on an empty stomach, after the elimination. Exercise before udvarthana and not after. Aftercare is as important—once you're done, rest for about 15 minutes and bathe with lukewarm water after an hour.

You don't need expensive powders for this practice. Even simple triphala, haritaki or reetha powder works well. If your aim is to beautify the complexion, you can also choose *musta* or anantmool powder, which helps enhance the complexion, whether rubbed topically or consumed with hot water as a tea. In traditional texts, there is also talk of brick powder being used for this method, but of course its best avoided. This practice isn't suitable for those with rosacea, as the extra rubbing inflames the skin even more. Additionally, those who have cuts, scrapes, psoriasis or eczema should not do this until their skin has recovered.

To do:

- Dust powder all over the body, avoiding the eyes, mouth and face. You could also dust powder part by part as you progress from the feet towards the face.
- Rub the soles and the top of the feet in a back-and-forth motion.

- The legs need to be rubbed in straight, vertical strokes against the direction of the hair. You know you're doing the correct movements when the hair stands up because of the opposing strokes.
- Rub the stomach and groin with both straight and circular strokes—clockwise and anti-clockwise. However, don't apply too much pressure on spots that feel tender.
- The chest must be rubbed with straight strokes towards the collarbone and circular strokes (both clockwise and anticlockwise) on the breasts.
- The sides of the body, back and arms to be rubbed in straight strokes aimed towards the heart.
- Udvarthana should not be done on the face and neck.

Detoxifying Powder

50 per cent horse gram (chana dal) powder
50 per cent triphala powder

Method:

Replace horse gram with barley powder if you have delicate, sensitive skin. You can use dry powders after an oil massage, or mix the them in a bit of oil. For detoxification, a warm oil such as mustard or sesame works best.

Beautifying Powder

50 per cent *nargarmotha* powder
30 per cent anantmool (sarsaparilla) powder
15 per cent rose petal powder
15 per cent mulethi (liquorice) powder

Method:

If you want to mix this with a fat, use a cooling oil like sweet almond or coconut, which is more suitable for beautifying the skin.

3

NABHI PURAN CHIKITSA

A fairly controversial concept, one that isn't really backed by science. But in our homes, we've reaped the benefits of rubbing herbs and spices over the belly as a common remedy for stomach discomfort, whether it's dry ginger or asafoetida for pain or bloating, or ghee in the navel to soften the skin. We know now that the skin has the ability to absorb nutrients. This ability has been utilised in Ayurveda, where oils that are prescribed as medicine are administered by massaging/pooling them within the navel.

The practice of *nabhi chikitsa* using the navel as a channel to disperse oils, herbs or/and essential oils. I like to do this every night before I sleep. It gives me a feeling of stability and has helped improve the quality of my skin and hair. Though it's debatable whether the technique works, as there isn't enough scientific evidence, there is anecdotal evidence to show that may help. It's also an immensely comforting evening ritual that can be done in the comfort of your bed.

Because the nabhi or navel lies right in the centre of the body, it is believed to have the ability to nurture you in all directions, whether it's up towards the head or down the legs. This central location is important as it is believed that if we nourish the centre, it will balance the rest of the body. We know that the navel is strategic during pregnancy and is key to the development of the foetus. The umbilical cord provides fresh, oxygenated blood to the infant and transfers the nutrient-depleted blood back to the placenta. The umbilical region also consists of the stomach and intestines, an area where food is converted into waste and energy. Even when we're stressed, we breathe into the navel to relax and breathe out the heaviness we don't need. This exchange happens naturally, so perhaps it's safe to assume that in both the physical and spiritual sense, our navel is a source of transformation.

The Folklore

From a metaphysical point of view, all 72,000 nadis or energy channels are connected to the navel. Therefore it is believed that nourishing it with certain oils can transfer the benefits all over the body. In meditation, the navel is considered to be the centre of consciousness—if the brain takes the attention outwards, focusing on the nabhi takes the attention inwards. Many meditation practices ask you to focus on the navel, which is considered to be the second brain. In acupuncture, the navel is called the Shenque point, CV8 or the spirit gate, which has connections with all the twelve principal meridians and internal organs.

In Japanese Zen meditation and martial arts, the *hara*, located just below the navel, is of great importance. In Zen meditation, practitioners are asked to breathe in and out of the hara (figuratively, of course), which bestows a sense of calmness. Not only is it considered to be the centre of energy for the body, it is also believed to have significant effects on mental, emotional and spiritual health. Even in oriental medicine, the navel is treated with moxibustion, a technique that applies heat by burning a candle of powdered mugwort herb to improve bodily functions.

In Ayurveda, an important marma point is situated behind the navel. It is called the *siras marma*—siras meaning blood vessels. It is believed that the blood vessels originate from this point, though anatomically it isn't so. The belly button is also the location of agni, which controls digestion and metabolism. It is believed that stimulating this point not only improves digestion but also helps detoxify the body. Additionally, it is the location of the solar plexus or the *manipura chakra*, that rules self-esteem and confidence.

Modern Revival

While there has been talk of a Pechoti gland believed to be behind the navel, supposedly connected to 70 million nerves. This elusive gland has regained popularity with CBD oil that many administer into the navel. While we don't know whether this Pechoti really exists, but it has been found that there are endocannabinoid receptors in the gut, which interact with nerves to aid digestion. Interestingly, an old study testing testosterone absorption suggests that absorption via the navel is almost as effective as an intravenous dose. So can we perhaps assume that there would be some amount of bioavailability via the navel, even though there isn't enough scientific evidence to support the practice of nabhi chikitsa?

My Experience

I started this practice with a healthy amount of scepticism. While I'd warm some oil or ghee to massage my feet, I'd dab a few drops into my belly button and give my abdomen a comforting rub during bedtime. In about a week or so, I noticed that my perpetually chapped lips (which required multiple applications of balm) weren't chapped anymore. The inside of my mouth felt smooth and my skin felt less dry than usual.

I use A2 cow's ghee for this ritual, which is supposed to calm the fiery pitta side of me, responsible for my greying hair and poor eyesight. Though I haven't noticed any changes to either yet, I live in the hope that ultimately this ritual may preserve my overall health. Though I choose ghee, different oils can be used for various purposes. It is believed that neem oil helps heal acne, castor oil reduces stomach problems, mustard oil detoxifies the body, almond oil beautifies the skin, sesame oil reduces joint pain and coconut oil reduces burning sensations and inflammation.

How to:

- Begin by warming your chosen oil. I like to transfer some ghee or oil into a small glass bottle which I place in a hot bowl of water to indirectly heat the fluid.

- Lie down in bed, pour 2-3 drops of the oil into your navel and hold it there for about a minute.
- Then gently massage it around the belly in circles, using gentle pressure.
- If you want to or have the time, repeat this a few more times, pouring warm oil every time and massaging it around.
- Alternatively, you can pour the oil into your navel and hold it there for about 25 minutes. You can even listen to a guided meditation at the same time.
- If you find holding the oil in your navel a bit messy, dip a ball of cotton into the oil and place it in your navel, especially if you're holding it for a longer duration.
- Use the same cotton wool or your fingers to spread the oil around the abdomen.
- Massage the abdomen gently with fingers and, if possible, either steam or place a hot-water bottle on the navel. This is useful to reduce bloating, as the main site of vata (the dosha of air and space, which causes bloating) is the large intestines.
- Your belly should feel warm by the end of the ritual. The best time to practise this is at night before bed.
- Do not practise this ritual if you have bacterial or fungal infection in the umbilical region.

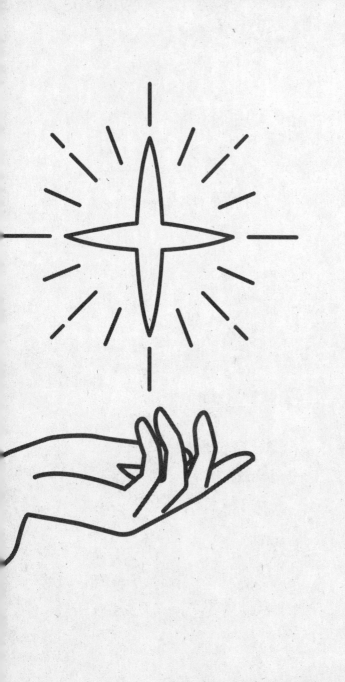

PILLAR II

✳

Heal

'We are healed of a suffering only by experiencing it to the full.'

—Marcel Proust, *In Search of Lost Time*

Healing begins with the acceptance that we are broken in the first place. We think of disease in black and white, but the reality is that ailments don't just appear out of a vacuum. Any condition is the ultimate manifestation of several internal breakdowns. It begins in the mind, increasing stress, elevating inflammation and eventually leading to chronic disease. The creation of disease and healing from it are both fairly nuanced activities. The diagnosis of a condition is its last sign, not the first. The body sends us several signals—chronic pain, tiredness, poor digestion, skin, hair and nail troubles—which are often ignored.

Compare the years of neglect that built up the disease to the amount of time you tried to get rid of it. If it took years to build, then it will take time to heal. You may take a pill to get rid of a symptom but that is only temporary. True recovery happens slowly, at various levels—mental, physical and emotional. Because the creation of disease happens due to multiple reasons, recovery too must be multipronged. People give up a remedy very soon because they think it didn't work.

Healing for me began with rituals—their stability, discipline, rigour and magic. Whether it was guided mediation, sound healing, journalling or massage, the stillness they provided helped me become aware of my inner dialogue. Just designating a certain amount of time was a signal for my subconscious that I was serious about getting better. And that's the thing with rituals—when you peel away the superstition and religion, they're just tools to refine, pacify, stimulate or heal the mind, body and spirit.

There is no doubt that traditional and modern medicine are both key to getting better and feeling great. There is no one practice that is the ultimate cure. Every healing protocol must be personalized to suit each individual's lifestyle, preferences and habits. Rituals make the process of healing very enjoyable. But for that, only choose what you like and what fits into your schedule.

Many ancient remedies were not grounded in science until recently but we knew they made us feel better. And it's not limited to just traditional practices. Solving the crossword, making your cup of coffee, applying skincare are all rituals when they're done with care. The rituals we have with animal companions, whether it's feeding them or taking them for a walk make us feel good. Now we also have proof that animal companions indeed reduce risk of mortality. In heart attack survivors who lived alone, the risk of death was reduced by 33 per cent if they kept a pet as compared to others who lived solitary lives. Another feel-good ritual is a hot bath before bed because it soothes the mind and helps us sleep better. Now studies explain exactly why: because our body temperatures peak in the afternoon and cool down as we approach bedtime, a warm bath brings out the heat towards the extremities, cooling the body and supporting the natural circadian rhythms.

We know that the things that make us feel good help us get better. So, is how we feel key to when we heal?

Our sense organs are very much involved in this process of healing. Watching a great movie, listening to music, eating a delicious meal and the human touch, all have the potential to transport us into a better, brighter space

Think about sound and its ability to change your mood. When the tempo is high, it makes us energetic, when low, more relaxed. In horror movies, sounds can be more terrifying than visuals. If it can scare you, it may also hold the potential to relax and heal you. Vibroacoustic therapy is when the vibration of sound is directly in touch with the body to work on a cellular level. It is believed by some practitioners that tuning forks held to the body can increase nitric oxide (a vasodilator also found in beetroot), which is excellent for cardiac health.

Then there is taste—it isn't just what you eat but how you eat it that determines how food affects your body. Taste, timing, posture and thorough mastication help it get broken down and digested by the body. Meals are also rituals. Eating with care and attention can maximize the impact of food on your body. Studies have shown that just the simple act of chewing food properly works like an 'oral meter' that helps us realize when we are actually satiated, thereby reducing the need to overeat.

The connection between feeling and healing becomes even more apparent in restorative practices including yin yoga, the

Nishi Health System exercises and the Alexander Technique. Breath, alignment and slow, restorative techniques are as valuable as high-intensity exercises. Slower workouts help us connect deeply to our body and also work at a much deeper level in terms of stretching the fascia and connective tissue. Longer holds without tensing the muscles in yin yoga ensure that poses increase flexibility deeply and gently.

To begin healing, stillness is important. The mind has the ability to both feed and starve disease, therefore it makes sense to sever mental and emotional ties to what made us unwell in the first place. But to peel away mental layers to finally recognize the real cause of suffering takes time. And even when you finally reach that last recognition, then what?

Sometimes I find that you can try everything but still not get better. In times like these, I found great value in acceptance and letting go. I know that things are bad and can become much worse. Instead of hoping for the best, I prepare for the worst. Sometimes our worst fears can materialize and at other times, they don't. But no matter what happens, we always find the strength to make it through. That is the beauty of human existence—we are born, we hope, we get hurt and no matter how bad it may be, eventually we all get through it.

1

SOUND HEALING

Everyone has different coping mechanisms. Some choose to sleep, others like to exercise and there are those (like me) who like to submerge themselves in work. But no matter how you rest and recover, it is safe to assume that everyone loves music. Sound has the ability to uplift the mood, it acts as a distraction and helps disconnect from stress. Music can make us feel energetic, melancholic, nostalgic, romantic or even gleeful. Sound, be it words or music, can be used as a weapon or a warm blanket. But our inner conversations matter much more than external sounds. Sound is both tangible and intangible. In fact, in yogic science the internal sounds of the body are of utmost importance to raise consciousness and connect with the energy of the universe.

The Origin of Sound

In the Indian context, music therapy comes from the school of nada yoga, which traces the origin of sound. According to this school of thought, sound is of two types—*ahata*, the struck sound and *anahata*, the unstruck sound. Most sounds we listen to are struck sounds, made by striking two objects, like the tongue and the mouth, the fingers and the guitar or drums etc. Indeed, these sounds are crucial as they can change our mood. However, for spiritual work, the most important sound is the unstruck sound, for instance, silent *japa* or mantra meditation, where we repeat the mantra mentally, feeling its vibrations without moving the mouth of the tongue.

Nada yoga literally means 'union through sound', as it is believed that the universe was first made of sound vibrations. One example of the universal sound is 'Om'. When we connect to the unstruck sound, whether it is through silent chanting of mantras or just focusing on the internal sounds of the body, it brings us closer to our own energetic frequencies. According to this ancient science, everything in the universe hums with its own rhythm. By connecting to these subtle sounds and frequencies, nada yogis become one with the universal energies. If you close your ears with your fingers, you will be able to listen to your own internal frequency, just like the sounds of waves in seashells.

Tuning Inwards

To tune into these subtle, inner sounds, nada experts suggest you listen to a piece of relaxing music like the sitar and *iktara* for about 10-15 minutes, then close your eyes and try to listen to the echo of these sounds. Do it daily if you have the inclination. The nada school also suggests that our bodies are made with five elements—earth, water, fire, air and space.

Out of these, the spatial element is the most primal because before everything took form, there was only space. Ancient texts suggest that this element is directly related to our sense of hearing. In fact, many years back, my healer told me that our sense of hearing, which incidentally is ruled by the space element, is the closest to the divine.

Interestingly, an old study found that listening to Mozart's 'Sonata for two pianos (K448)' led to better spatial reasoning. The Mozart effect is a term that was coined as a direct result of this study, where it was believed that listening to Mozart can boost brain power, even though the study only talks about boosting spatial reasoning and that too for a period of 15 minutes. Still, whether it's boosting creativity or soothing the mind, the therapeutic effects of sound cannot be denied. All cultures around the world have their own variation of sound healing. Tibetans have their singing bowls, the Japanese have their *sahari orin* (Buddhist bells) that are said to purify the environment with sound, and we have our own set of Hindustani classical instruments.

Ayurveda has several theories based on sound and its impact on the doshas. For instance, a sturdy, kapha-dominant person can listen to 'hard' music, which could mix several types of instruments, tempos and frequencies. Compare that to a more delicate, easily disturbed vata personality, who can get drained by the same sounds and will find music that is softer, smoother and unidimensional more healing. It's worth noting that as we age, the vata element increases in the body, which, among other things, also makes the body drier. Therefore, the type of music that we found energizing in youth becomes draining as we advance in years.

51

Rooted in Tradition

Ragas are a great example of sounds to suit the mood. For instance, the optimistic tempo of raga *bhatiyar* is perfect for dawn as compared to the solemn raga *marwah*, which is suited for dusk. Then there is raga chikitsa, used for its therapeutic effects on the body. A paper exploring the effect of ragas by capturing EEG signals in the brain lists the ten parent ragas and their usage: *bhairav* and *bhairavi* are both morning ragas, the former played at daybreak. *Asavari* is a romantic morning raga, while *bilawal*, played at the same time, conveys joy. If meditation is part of your a.m. ritual, then raga *todi* bestows a meditative atmosphere. *Kafi* can be played at any time for its *shringar*/romantic mood, while *purvi* is an afternoon raga for serenity. Among evening ragas, there's the aforementioned marwah for its ascetic mood, bilawal for joy, *kalyan* and *khamaj* for peace and happiness.

There are also ragas with very specific effects on the brain. For instance, raga *nilambari* can aid sleep while raga *bhupali* serves as an invitation to wake up. *Bilahari* helps alleviate melancholy and *sama* raga is said to reduce anxiety. However, alternative therapies must be treated as part of the whole line of treatment, which includes consulting a mental health professional.

Mantras are another example of healing with sounds. It is believed that when mantras are chanted verbally, they purify the environment. When chanted silently, they work from within, healing the individual or the inner, etheric body. But the science of mantras must be studied and practised under an experienced teacher. Typically, a mantra is highly individualized and recommended by a teacher.

Still, within the sphere of sound healing, I have found guided mantra meditations that bestow a sense of peace. For instance, there's chakra meditation, with repetitions of various a syllables assigned to every chakra—'lam' for the root, 'vam' for the sacral, 'ram' for the solar plexus, 'yam' for the heart, 'ham' for the heart and 'om' for both the third eye and the crown.

The Modern Relevance of Sound

Music can transport us wherever we want, we don't need need research to prove this. It can make us energetic, relaxed, joyful or melancholic. Lullabies put babies to sleep. Celebrations are incomplete without dance and music. Sounds, words, melodies have the ability to build or destroy the mood. Today we're living in an age where our senses are heavy with overstimulation—be it the eyes, tired with never-ending visuals, or ears loaded with sounds of traffic, airplanes, loudspeakers, sirens, and chatter. In fact, noise annoyance is now recognized as an important environment stressor, linked to depression and anxiety. On the contrary, natural sounds have been proven to increase focus and feelings of relaxation. It's no surprise then that most of us who live in the city and spend time connected to our mobiles and tablets are anxious.

One way or another, our brain is always working, primarily with four main frequencies. The first is the beta wave, at 15 to 40 cycles a second. This is when our mind is highly engaged. If you're making a speech, you're in high beta. Then come the alpha waves at 9 to 14 cycles a second. This is when we take a break from work, sip a cup of tea or go for a walk. The third is the theta wave with 5 to 8 cycles a second. We're in theta state when we're daydreaming, running, painting or meditating. Sometimes when we're in the shower we get a brilliant idea. This happens when the mind is in the theta frequency. The last is delta at 1 1/2 to 4 cycles a second. This happens when we sleep.

Music is known to increase alpha and decrease beta activity over time. For instance, a popular modality for sound healing are binaural beats. These are supposed to create an auditory illusion with two different frequencies in each ear, giving the impression of a third rhythmic beat. For instance, if two different beats of close frequencies are presented at the same time, say 400 hz to the left ear and 440 hz to the right, the difference between the two (in this case 40 hz) is the frequency perceived by the brain. When this happens, it is believed that the neurons start sending signals at the same rhythm as this beat, increasing feelings of relaxation.

Scientific reports on this are mixed, even though many people report feeling relaxed after listening to binaural beats. For every study that refutes sound healing, there's another that supports it. These findings aren't just limited to binaural beats. There is a report that claims the sound of drums helps reduce substance abuse as part of the complementary therapy. Another says that the sound of Tibetan bowls helps reduce tension, anger and fatigue. But can we only listen to sound and eliminate anger and worry? Alternative therapies are best used as supportive remedies that are part of a whole line of treatment. However, they can always be used just to take a quick break and destress the mind. Of course, becoming a nada yogi requires years of practice and learning. And any type of deep meditation must always be learnt in person with a teacher.

But that isn't to say there are no benefits. Sound can and must be utilized to feel better. Listening to a favourite song always makes us feel good. But just as favourite songs differ from one person to another, so does sound healing. Some may enjoy an evening raga, while others prefer delta meditation before going to bed. Some chant silent mantras, while others enjoy the sound of rain.

I like sound healing because it is also the easiest meditative activity. Most forms of meditation have a technique which can be mentally exhausting for some. But sound healing is never exhausting. All you need is a sound you like; then just sit or lie back and listen to it.

Sound healing in daily life:

1. Use it to take a break. Listen to your choice of music/ nature sound/binaural beat to energize yourself during a late afternoon slump.
2. Use it to go to sleep. If you feel a little out of sorts, you could listen to the chakra mantras before you go to bed.
3. Use it to energize yourself in the morning. Listen to up-tempo music or a morning raga.
4. You can listen to sound in any manner. If you want something relaxing and meditative, listen to it in bed. Lie on your back with arms and legs spread apart, and listen to a healing meditation or even your favourite piece of music.

5. Sound healing as passive meditation can help you disconnect from thought without putting in too much effort.

6. We know that music is personal, therefore healing with sound is also highly individualized. Make a choice based on your preferences, not your friend's or family member's. What they find soothing could be disturbing for you and vice versa.

2

THE ART OF EATING

We're living at a time when the word 'superfood' is part of everyday language. We're reasonably knowledgeable about herbs that boost immunity, we have recipes for detoxifying smoothies and understand how to count our macros in a meal. But despite all the knowledge, herbs and superfoods at hand, we're still not getting better. For some, especially those with chronic disease, it feels like our bodies reject the nutrition that we so carefully plan and consume. Could it be that we stop looking at food as something that needs to be weighed, measured and counted? Is the definition of nutrition only limited to the food we eat or does it go far beyond what's on the plate?

The truth is that it's not just what's on our plate, but how we eat, the timing, posture and our relationship with food, that must all be considered as a part of nutrition. We all have a million things on our to-do lists, which is why we're always rushed. Mealtimes are regularly sacrificed in a hurry: we skip meals, eat quickly, at the wrong time, because work takes precedence over well-being. But sacrificing meals and staying disconnected to food decreases its positive impact. Because how we eat is as important as what we eat.

1. Chew Well

Ayurveda recommends chewing each morsel 30 to 50 times, but most of us don't chew our food thoroughly. We know now that chewing thoroughly prevents overeating and helps release gut hormones that signal secretion of enzymes leading to better digestion and absorption of nutrients. From a spiritual point of view, it helps us connect better with food, therefore our bodies accept the nourishment provided.

2. Sit Straight

How we sit while we eat and what we do after meals also affects digestion. Slouching over during and after meals leads to poor gut health—just think of how you're compressing your organs. When we hunch, slouch or lie down after a meal, it can increase bloating and stomach distress. When the spine is curved forward it contracts the abdomen, which means there's less space for the food to move around. This contracted abdomen also sends stomach acid in the wrong direction.

3. Walk After a Meal

Poor posture during and after meals also affects how the food passes through the digestive tract. We don't even need evidence for this. Just eat a meal and lie down for a nap. See how that feels versus when you eat a meal and walk for 10 minutes. Ayurveda recommends we walk at least 100 steps after meals for better digestion. Try walking those steps and you'll find that the difference in bloating and digestion is remarkable.

4. Don't Eat Till You're Full

Another simple food rule suggested by traditional sciences is to stop eating when the stomach is two thirds full. In Japan, the phrase '*hara hachi bu*' meaning eat till you're 80 per cent full, originated in Okinawa, an island, known to have a high percentage of centenarians. It takes time for the brain to register that the stomach is full. Eat slowly and only till where you're just about satisfied. This helps prevent the bloated feeling after a meal, which often leads to abdominal discomfort.

5. Look Beyond Nutrition

If you look at the food habits of people who live in blue zones (areas where people live the longest), you'll find that it's all balancing daily practices. They primarily eat a plant-based diet with vegetables, legumes, oils and grains that grow naturally in their region. The diet is low in processed food but contains bits of fish and meat that are used mostly as condiments to flavour the food. They walk a lot as part of their daily routine, and not like us city folk, who limit it to just an hour in the evening. They fast weekly, take daily naps (shorter than 30 minutes), and have healthy social and familial connections. Therefore, it isn't just about the amount of nutrients in food but also balancing the various aspects of wellness—physical, emotional and spiritual.

Food and Circadian Rhythms

In 2020, the world shut down. The lockdown either perfected your daily routine, or destroyed it. I've always had a changing relationship with wellness—either I'm in my sattvic phase, sleeping before 10 p.m., waking up at dawn—or going to bed and waking up late. I went through both phases in the lockdown. When I felt emotionally settled, I was disciplined. Of course, it's difficult to follow a strict routine when the mind is disturbed. But going to bed later disturbed my sleep quality making me feel lethargic later in the day. Being disciplined requires and provides mental stability so it's a bit of a catch-22 situation. Still, it's a no-brainer that by just following the circadian rhythms improves sleep quality, energy levels and digestion.

Traditional Body Clock

In TCM, the health of the liver is connected to the health of the rest of the organs. When it functions well, it regulates chi (the life force within the body), facilitates the process of digestion and absorption, regulates the flow of blood and manages emotions. The peak time for the liver to work according to the Chinese clock is between 1 a.m. and 3 a.m. TCM textbooks, such as *Healing with Whole Foods* by Paul Pitchford, recommend that meals be taken as further away from this time of the liver. Because for it to work properly all digestion must be complete.

A simple meal of grains and legumes takes 3 hours in the stomach and another 3 hours in the intestines. In Ayurveda, it is advised that meats and fish be eaten in the day because of their long digestion time—red meat takes up to 8 hours to be digested, chicken 6 hours and fish 4 hours. This is why our traditional system of *do waqt ki roti* instead of three meals in the day works better for smooth functioning of the internal organs. The last meal of the day must always be the lightest, so that it can get adequately digested before 'liver time'.

Ayurvedic practitioners also recommend eating grains at lunch because around noon, the metabolic fire or agni is at its peak. From the TCM perspective, if the meal is eaten with an hour of noon, it falls during the heart/mind time. This means that our intuition is better, what and how much to eat is clearer, therefore food decisions are wiser.

But the biggest rule for eating intuitively is to eat simply, and only when hungry. Overstimulating food such as a bag of chips or a juicy burger are designed to make the mouth water even when you're not hungry. This is why partaking in simple meals is very important, because they help change your palate.

Eat right:

- Sit straight when you eat.
- Walk 100 steps after a meal.
- Drink water sparingly during a meal.

- Do not drink cold water/chilled drinks with a meal as it can make saturated fats congeal.
- Stay connected to your food, avoid scrolling on the phone or watching television.
- Eat your biggest meal at noon.
- Synchronize mealtimes with circadian rhythms.
- Keep dinner light.
- Ayurveda recommends you eat sweets at the beginning of the meal to feel satiated. Or keep dessert to be eaten in between meals as a snack.
- Ideal mealtimes are: breakfast between 7 and 9 a.m., lunch between 11 a.m. and 1 p.m., dinner between 4 and 7 p.m.
- According to TCM, if you're eating high protein foods, keep them at the beginning of the meal so that they get broken down with the stomach acids that haven't yet been used.
- Keep meals simple. This means one type of grain and one protein. Mixing too many grains and proteins in a meal makes it harder to digest.
- Sprouting grains, legumes and seeds makes them more digestible, and increases their nutritional content.
- Both TCM and Ayurveda recommend cooked foods for those with weak digestion.
- Practising gratitude towards food, either by praying before a meal or being attentive towards it, improves our relationship with what we eat.

3

JOURNALLING

Writing is therapeutic for me, whether it's work or writing in my diary, especially when there's something that I need to unravel about myself.

Journalling is extremely relaxing for me, because I don't need to be prolific. I write whatever comes to my mind, the words flow easily, without judgement, because they are for my eyes only. It is one way to see myself clearly and think freely.

Journalling gives me clarity of thought. We always advise people to look at a situation through a third person's perspective. Writing is one way to do that because it takes the thoughts out of your mind and on to paper. When thoughts are written in black and white, it provides more clarity than when they're just floating in your mind. Sometimes it's like letting go and at others, it provides you the material to resolve something methodically.

When you journal regularly, it's interesting to go back a couple of years to see how far you've come. You may have not even come very far, or the written words don't matter to you anymore, but they could bring closure and a sense of moving on. Also, the words remind what you must never go back to again. We psyche our minds to shut out painful memories and choose the ones that we want to remember. This is a coping mechanism, but the goal of journalling is not just to resist painful memories and grasp at positive ones, but to acknowledge all memories and their accompanying emotions.

When journalling is done in this manner, then neuroplasticity, which is the ability of our brains to change in both form and function, can happen as the synapses (the connection between neurons) get more sensitive, and new neurons grow when used repeatedly, for instance, when we recall a memory. But the thing with our mind is that it adds a subjective tint to our memories, by subconsciously factoring who we are, and what we feel and believe at the time of recollection. So every time we recall something, it is changed and more charged.

Because of this, journalling also serves as a reality check. Whether it's an incident or your feelings, there's no denying that something or someone made you feel a certain way when it's been documented on paper. Therefore, journalling helps to track our patterns of thinking, its improvements and changes over time.

How to Begin

Writing our most intimate thoughts can be intimidating, even for the most seasoned writer. So how does one write the truth and can it be easy? Like anything else, writing also improves with practice. Those who haven't exercised this muscle may feel a little stuck but when this happens, you may want to introspect for a few moments beforehand. There's no need to rush into it. Explore what or who made you happy/ sad, what exactly happened, what is it that you wanted to do differently. If you feel particularly stuck, then doodling, drawing or watercolours can take the place of words.

You could also pick one affirmation and write it down every day. One of my favourite affirmations is 'Every day in every way I get better and better.' I like this because this applies to getting better in any aspect of your life, be it health, work, confidence or your spiritual journey. As you write, imagine yourself healing and improving. This too is therapeutic.

Another way to look at journaling is a way to explore yourself. Sometimes other people know more about us than we do. It could be because we're always thinking of what others are thinking, which is why we're afraid to express ourselves and put our needs last that causes a disconnect with our true nature. In this case, journaling is a way to get to know yourself better. 'What are the qualities that I like in people?' 'What will I never tolerate?' 'What do boundaries mean for me?' 'Why do I find it difficult to say no?' It's easy to become more cognizant about your likes and dislikes when they're listed down clearly.

The good thing about writing therapy is that it is comes with minimal side effects, and over time, can give insights about patterns that could go unnoticed when thoughts remain in the mind. However, in rare cases, it could be detrimental for those who have no support. If writing about traumatic events causes severe distress, it is advisable to contact a mental health professional. For therapeutic benefits, it is recommended to write 15–20 minutes a day. However, if you intend to cultivate writing as a ritual for a lifetime, start slow by writing for a few minutes and slowly build up every day.

Writing has always helped me release something—be it mental clutter thrown on papers as a to-do list or writing about a deeply emotional experience and deleting the file immediately to erase any record of dark thoughts. I write on my laptop, make bullet points on my phone, I have a special silk-lined journal for my experiences. It's this journal that I turn to when I want guidance. Just flipping back a few pages reminds me of previous experiences that I'd forgotten. Sometimes they're a reminder of a dark past and at other times, they're a reminder to show how much I've progressed.

Sometimes, when I have nothing to write, I'll write about how I envision my future or how I want to transform as a person. When I was younger, we were told that too much reading and writing would run our eyesight. But today, as we stare with rapt fascination at our screens, doom-scrolling and unable to stop, journaling provides a safe shelter. It's immensely private, healing, thought-provoking and transformative. If you're the kind of person who doesn't want the spiritual mumbo-jumbo of a yogic practice, but still wants to calm an overactive mind, try writing in a journal to unburden yourself.

Writing Pointers

- Don't write for anyone else, only write for yourself.
- If the task overwhelms you, answer a question: what feelings do I have that I want to recognize today? What do I hate today? What do I love today? Where do I want

to be in a year? What's bothering me? The pros and cons of a job or a relationship.

- It could just be a factual record, such as what you ate in a day.

- Just like any other ritual, writing is all about practice. The more you do it, the easier it flows.

- Write for as long as you want to; for therapeutic benefits, 15-20 minutes are recommended.

- Always mark the dates on a fresh note in your journal. This helps you track your progress and keep records.

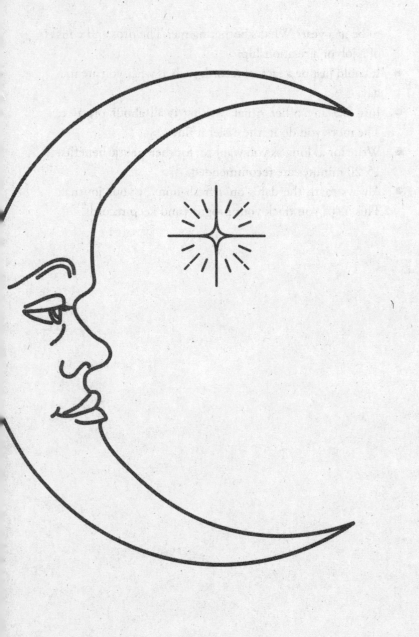

PILLAR III

✳

Rest

'We are going to the moon that is not very far. Man has so
much farther to go within himself.'

—Anaïs Nin, *The Diary of Anaïs Nin*

The problem with sleep is that we expect it to be
instantaneous—close your eyes and it will come. But
we cannot switch from active to rest mode in one fell swoop.
Our minds, emotions and body all need to be prepared
during the evening for relaxation, just like we prepare in the
morning for activity. Some people avoid caffeine during in
the afternoon, others skip an afternoon nap to ensure they
feel sleepy at night. Either way, it is up to you to find a
personalized routine that will help you get a good night's
rest. Because we cannot expect sleep to come just because we
want it to. If you want to rest well, you have to prioritize and
prepare for it.

Perhaps it is considered futile in the modern world
because we don't really 'do' anything when asleep. Tangible
results from productivity are of high value, therefore activities
such as exercising, working, researching, studying or even
scrolling on social media take precedence. But the reality is
that qualitative hours of sleep enhance the body's function,
priming it to be more productive during the day.

Sleep converts short-term memory into long-term memories. It erases superfluous information that may clutter the nervous system and cause undue stress, thereby providing emotional stability. Quality sleep regulates glucose levels and boosts immunity.

Interestingly, the inner world of your body is working hard to detoxify and repair itself, even though you may be immobile while you sleep. The brain is active when you're at rest, storing memories and getting rid of toxic waste. The body releases various hormones during the different stages of sleep, therefore a lack of it poorly effects the endocrine system. When you're active, the body needs to support all outward functions such as movement and digestion. It's only when you're completely at rest does it get the chance to work inwards.

High energy levels, better cognitive ability, heart health, immunity and reduced inflammation are just a few among the multitude of benefits that are bestowed by sleep. People who sleep well lead healthier, happier and longer lives. If you're a doer, you can enhance the quality of every activity just by replenishing the body's reserves at night. Sleep is the best anti-depressant, the best supplement, the magic brew that makes everything better. It isn't an occasional booster shot, but must be prioritized and planned for every single day.

Wellness is all about balancing the opposites—to eat and fast, work and play, activity and rest. We work so we can earn the means to live our aspired lives. But when you have a high-stress job, there is a chance you spend a substantial chunk of those earnings on health. Rest reduces stress and inflammation, which means that even if it can't completely prevent disease, it can certainly reduce its severity.

If you want qualitative sleep, you must begin preparation a couple of hours before bed. During this time, every mental and physical activity must be intended towards rest. This means minimal stimulation, be it books, movies or podcasts. Enjoy winding down the day, soothe yourself with healing spices and herbs infused into a tea. Practise breathwork that helps you disconnect from the day so that the mind is calm before bed.

Sometimes, even (or especially) when the body is exhausted, the mind can keep us up at night. I find that the worst, most fatalistic thoughts come through after dark. Ordinary worries about unfinished assignments, or imaginative fantasies about disease and disaster, are all projected by a fertile mind. It's difficult to rein in the disturbing chain of thoughts. I try to distract myself by reading a book or a phone call, but when I feel inclined, I like to observe these thoughts—where they come from and where they're leading. To do this, I find that using a technique always results in a calmer mind, as opposed to a freestyle dip into my mind, which ends up entangling my thoughts even more.

Evenings are a wonderful time to unwind by tuning into the esoteric world of mantras, guided meditation and breathwork. The breath is in fact the best tool for mind control. Just like it can be used to energize the body in the morning, it can also be channelized to calm the mind at the end of the day. Breathwork helps the body switch from the sympathetic to the parasympathetic nervous system—the former rules activity, while the latter rules rest and restoration. Because of this calming effect, pranayama has been proven to reduce blood pressure and improve sleep. Whether it's via longer exhalations or breathing into the abdomen, pranayama offers several practices that help you rest better.

Bedtime rituals are of utmost importance because they send signals to the body and mind that it is time to relax. Relaxing massages, soothing beverages or calming meditative techniques work in a synchronistic manner, taking you one step after another into a state of complete rest. For me, my nightly face massage marks the cut-off time for activity. After I've worked my skin with the energy and intention to relax, it seems unnecessary to let anything come into my sacred space, least of all social media.

A friend once told me that the beginning of the day is about hope, while the end of the day must be about gratitude. When we begin, we must always do so with the expectation that things will go well and when we end, for our own peace of mind, it is prudent to appreciate what went right. While it is essential to critically assess what went wrong during the day, your bed isn't the place to do it. Because even on the worst day, there is always something that went right.

1

PREPARING FOR REST

Sleep, like love, happens naturally, when it's least expected. It's never forced, which is why overthinking makes it all the more elusive. Therefore, it is critical to ensure that the body and mind are completely relaxed by the time you go to bed. Planning and preparing may sound complicated, but it merely implies that you need to make relaxation a priority.

There's no point reading a thriller, scrolling on social media or watching a highly stimulating mini-series before bed, because they energize and engage the mind instead of relaxing it. In addition to screen time being upsetting/exciting, the light from your phone or tablet also suppresses melatonin, a hormone that becomes activated after dark and signals to the body that it's time to rest.

Of course, not everyone has the privilege to avoid high-energy conversations before bed, but we do have a choice to keep the phone away. Because the chatter of thousands of people on social media is infinitely more disturbing than engaging with family at home. For many of us, the phone has become an escape, a distraction or something to do. Let's not forget that for most of us, our screen time is a few hours every day. So, we all have the time to squeeze out several minutes to practise a ritual that—mentally and physically—removes the baggage that may clog the mind.

Elevate Your Feet

Putting your feet up after a long day is more than just an idiom. In both traditional and modern sciences, lifting your feet helps aid relaxation. Most of us have sedentary jobs, because of which the circulation becomes sluggish. As we are seated for hours at a time, it can lead to problems such as blood clots, swollen feet and ankles. Therefore, by elevating the feet above the chest level, we can direct all that blood back towards the heart and brain, releasing pressure from the lower limbs.

When we reverse the gravitational pull, the veins have to work less to push the blood towards the heart. But being upside down has myriad benefits, especially in yoga. The practice of inversions, for instance, is said to convert sexual energy into spiritual energy. When we're inverted, the breathing becomes slower and the mind is more relaxed and therefore, less excited. Inversions also help improve meditative practices, but they must only be learnt from a teacher. A seasoned guru will teach you how not to put pressure on your neck and shift it towards the shoulders. However, gentler variations of inversions can be practised safely at home and will help you feel relaxed and comforted after a long day.

Supported Vipritkarni

The gentler variation of the full shoulder stand, the *vipritkarni* is restorative for the body. To make it even more relaxing, you can use the wall for support. This is a wonderful pose after a stressful day or an especially hard workout. While shoulder stands always require a warm-up, you can get into this supported version without one and it is guaranteed to make you feel good. The legs above the wall give you a sense of balance as the blood and lymphatic fluids start flowing in the opposite direction, which bestows a restful feeling.

While you can do this towards the end of the day, you can also get into this pose during the afternoon during an energy slump. The only caveat is that you must have eaten lunch about 2 hours prior, a fruit about an hour to 45 minutes beforehand or juice/water 20 minutes earlier.

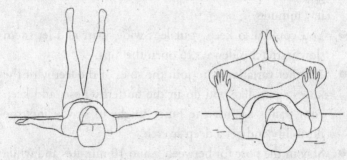

Variation 1 of supported vipritkarni   Variation 2 of supported vipritkarni

- Roll out a yoga mat, a thick sheet, a carpet or a dhurrie close to the wall.

- Bring your hips as close to the wall as possible and then gently swing your legs up. You will need to wiggle your hips forward to bring them in contact with the wall, so that the body can be in an 'L' shape with your back on the mat and legs up the wall.

- If you feel a strain on your hamstrings, keep a little bit of distance between your hips and the wall. If you find there to be some strain on your lower back, place a cushion or bolster (horizontally) underneath your back, right under your tailbone. You could also keep a small cushion underneath your neck to support your head, if you feel the need.

- Keep your legs and knees straight if your hamstrings are flexible; if not, keep the legs apart and knees gently bent—the latter variation is more relaxing.

- If you want to open your hamstrings and feel more grounded, place a bolster on the soles of your feet for a few minutes.

- You could also keep your legs wide apart and let them slowly stretch sideways to open the hips.

- Another variation is to join the soles of the feet with the knees apart, like you do in the butterfly pose, and keep your palms against the inner thighs to slowly increase flexibility and get a deep stretch.

- Stay in the pose for between 5 and 10 minutes and while you're here, breathe deeply. Focus on a minimum of 25 deep breaths, tracing the movement of your breath from the nostrils to the throat, down the chest and stomach till the pelvic floor. Then trace the movement of the exhale in the same manner from the pelvis till the nostril.

- You can even do this pose in your bed with the feet up the wall.

2

BEVERAGES

There's nothing more comforting than a pre-bed beverage. Whether it's warm milk with cocoa or a steaming cup of herbal tea, this ritual is immensely relaxing and underlines the end of the day. I enjoy the feeling of warmth in my belly and also find that certain beverages like triphala tea give me a feeling of lightness before bed. Other times, when I've had a particularly exhausting day, I choose a more restorative drink such as turmeric milk that gives me a feeling of replenishment before I sleep. The ritual remains the same but I tweak it regularly, changing it according to the seasons and my body's needs.

I usually go to bed with a mug of hot herbal tea in one hand and a small cup of hot water in another. In this cup of hot water, I immerse a small bottle of ghee to warm up, which takes barely a few moments. Then I put a few drops of the warm, melted ghee into my navel and rub some on the soles of my feet. By then, my tea has cooled down to a drinkable temperature. I sip this tea slowly, usually reading something non-stimulating, like a book on health/wellness/spirituality. In fact, reading a book on sleep makes me feel most sleepy.

By the time the tea is finished, my eyes are rolling back into their sockets, and I'm ready for a good night's rest.

My favourite book to read before bed is *Why We Sleep* by Matthew Walker. In his book—which I have extensively consulted to write these chapters—Walker says that humans are the only animals who forcefully keep themselves awake. Whether it's to watch a mini-series, go for a party, wait for a call, but mostly for no good reason, we always delay sleep. Even though most activities can be postponed till the next day, we force ourselves into a state of wakefulness. This is why bedtime hygiene is important. Daily rituals help streamline your evening instead of getting pulled into a vortex of stimulation.

Milk Instead of Caffeine

Coffee must be avoided the afternoon onwards as it can take up to 7 hours for it to be metabolized by the body. Evening beverages must be taken either for better sleep, digestion or to calm the mind. Whether you opt for a nostalgia-inducing a mug of hot cocoa or a new-age moon milk, if they're made with good quality dairy, they will enhance sleep. Milk contains tryptophan, an amino acid that gets metabolized into niacin, serotonin and melatonin, which collectively help you sleep better. Other sources of tryptophan include tuna, chicken, turkey, oats, nuts, seeds and chocolate.

Restorative Teas

The second amino acid to aid sleep is L-Theanine, which promotes relaxation at night and attentiveness during the day. Animal studies show that it increases the production of serotonin and dopamine along with GABA (gamma amino butyric acid), all of which are calming neurotransmitters. It has been found that a combination of L-theanine and GABA decreases the time it takes to go to sleep and increases its duration. Both L-Theanine and GABA are found in green and black tea, which is why (despite the caffeine content) drinking a cup of tea is infinitely more calming than coffee. However, if you choose to drink tea before bedtime, choose the decaffeinated variety. You can also drink teas with mulethi (yashti madhu) or tulsi as they help calm the mind (for directions see pg. 100 in SUN).

Ayurvedic Herbs

Traditional medicines prescribe several herbs for better sleep. Among these, *tagara*, jatamansi, *ashwagandha*, brahmi and tulṣi are the most calming for the mind. Tagara and jatamansi both come from the valerian family and are used specifically for sleep. While both bestow a sense of calm, tagara may be better than jatamansi in initiation of sleep, its quality and duration. This is because tagara contains a higher percentage of valepotriates, which are the active ingredient in valerian, that make it a potent sedative. They work by preventing the breakdown of GABA (a neurotransmitter mentioned above). Consult your doctor before you take any ayurvedic herbs if you're pregnant. In fact, both jatamansi and tagara must be taken in consultation with an ayurvedic physician, who can help you with the correct dosage.

Let's also not forget the ever-popular ashwagandha, which helps strengthen the nerves and reduce cortisol, the stress hormone, in the body. This root is prized because at one end, it helps increase mental and physical stamina and on the other, it also helps improve sleep quality and reduce insomnia. It can, however, be drying, therefore I prefer to take it with a bit of animal fat, i.e., either a teaspoon with a cup of milk or with another teaspoon of ghee. If you're vegan, take it with a cup of hot water.

3

BREATHWORK FOR RELAXATION

When we're stressed, we often forget to breathe. We all know that breathing deeply leads to a calmer mind, but do you know why that happens? A recently discovered neural pathway in the brain, was found to adjust various levels of emotions depending on how we breathe. In our physical body, slow, deep breathing lowers blood pressure, reduces free radical load and strengthens the respiratory muscles. If you've practised pranayama, you don't need a scientific study to tell you that it helps lighten the mind—you know it by experience.

Before going to bed, when the brain is buzzing and heavy with the happenings of the day, breathwork can help release excessive thoughts to a certain degree. Of course, breathwork for the evening is entirely different from what we practise in the morning. If sunrise practices are done after sunset, it would lead to an increase in energy, which is best avoided if you wish to sleep at night. The ground rules remain the same—the spine must be straight, and the stomach must be empty as you practise. This means 2 hours after a full meal and 1 hour after a snack.

You could also choose to do the evening pranayama between the hours of 3 and 5 p.m. According to Ayurveda, this is vata time, governed by the energies of air and space, the same dosha that dominates the early morning hours (3-5 a.m.), making these hours perfect for meditative work. But if you wish to practise it before bed, do it, because it will help you release your thoughts. I sometimes like to meditate just before bedtime. This isn't recommended because meditation is never perfect when one is sleepy. In fact, depending on your practice, some types of meditation can even energize you before bed. But I sometimes do it as it puts me in the mood to sleep. Sure, my meditation may not be attentive or perfect, but at least I rest well.

Brahmari

Translated literally, *brahmari* means humming bee, which is the sound you hear when you practise this pranayama. The internalized buzzing sound reverberates through the body and helps break the tempo of a running mind. It helps reduce heart rate, blood pressure and stress levels, thereby making the mind calmer. If you're feeling anxious, practise this for 5 minutes to break the chain of disturbing thoughts. This is best practised early morning or late at night, though it can also be done at any time whenever you're anxious, overthinking or stressed.

1. Sit either in a comfortable cross-legged position or on a chair with both feet on the floor. Do not cross your legs if seated on the chair. Also, never practise this lying down.

2. Close both ears with your thumbs. Makes sure all the muscles in your face are soft and loose. You front teeth should be slightly apart.

3. Inhale all the way into your belly and exhale making an extended 'hum' sound. Don't over-exhale—the sound should be even and continuous. Also, you shouldn't need to gulp the next inhale.

4. If you can, keeping your eyes closed, focus on the point between your brows.

5. If you want a variation, you can also replace the 'hum' with an 'om' sound, keeping your lips lightly closed.

6. Repeat 5 to 7 times.

7. Avoid if you have an ear infection.

Did you know?

Long, sharp exhales calm the nervous system. Therefore, focusing on longer exhales is a great practice to prepare the body for rest.

Belly Breathing

When we're stressed, our natural instincts guide us to breathe deeply. Inhaling and exhaling into the belly is a more relaxed state of breathing. This is how children breathe but as we grow older, our breaths become shallower. It's only when we consciously try to relax ourselves that we breathe deep into the belly. When I used to teach yoga, I'd ask students to breathe not just into the belly but deep into the pelvic floor.

When we're always in a state of stress, I find that we tighten and clench the entire pelvis, including the glutes. Breathing as deeply as possible helps release the tightness in the abdomen and pelvis.

Sometimes I'd also add visualization along with deep abdominal beathing right in the beginning of class. I would ask students to imagine their breath to be a large fishing net that would shore up negative emotions with an inhale and throw them out with an exhale. This would work as a temporary release to help them focus on the class. You could try this visualization to help eliminate stressful thoughts.

However, with deep-seated anxiety, depression and/or sleep problems, it is essential to consult a mental health professional or a somnologist. But even then, deep breathing can work as a complementary therapy to aid relaxation as it helps reduce levels of cortisol (the stress hormone) and could help you sleep better.

- Lie down on your back with a thin pillow under your head, keeping your legs apart, your left hand on your chest and right hand on your belly.
- Inhale slowly and deeply, first into your chest, then upper and lower belly, and last into your pelvis. If you're clenching your glutes, unclench them.
- Breathe out from your pelvis, lower and upper abdomen, chest and exhale through the mouth.
- Feel the rise and fall of your belly.
- Breathe only as deeply as you're comfortable. Both the inhale and exhale should be smooth and not laboured.
- Start with 10 deep breaths and move up to 25.

- Like any other pranayama, this too must be practised on an empty stomach.
- You can add a visualization if you like—either utilizing the breath as a giant fishnet or imagining it as a source of golden light filling up the body. You can also do this along with sound healing, using one of the Solfeggio frequencies.

4-7-8 Breath

This is another technique, which helps reduce levels of cortisol. In fact, the three pranayamas mentioned in this chapter can be practised one after another—brahmari while seated, belly breathing lying down, and finally this breath right at the end. Dr Andrew Weil, integrative medicine practitioner and teacher, devised this ratio of breath to be practised regularly, which (over time) relaxes the mind and helps you ease into sleep.

- Lie down or sit straight. Keep your facial features and mouth relaxed.
- Place the tip of the tongue gently behind the upper front teeth without tightening the mouth, tongue or jaw.
- Inhale to the count of 1-4.
- Hold the breath to the count of 1-7.
- Exhale slowly to the count of 1-8.
- Do 4 cycles to begin and then increase the number. Practise this twice a day to feel more relaxed over time.

Physiological Sighs

The pattern of two inhales through the nose followed by a long exhale through the mouth, similar to when we cry. Sighing helps relieve tension in those undergoing stress, therefore this technique may help relax the body and offload tension.

4

SLEEP POSTURE

If you're lucky, you spend a third of your life sleeping. Unfortunately, most of our attention is diverted to our waking hours, even though most of us are severely sleep-deprived. A good night's rest isn't time wasted. To say that sleep is a little death would only be accurate in the sense that when you do sleep deeply, it is like being born again. But, sleep is far from death because it feeds the brain. When well-rested, the brain is able to retain new learnings, boost memory while at the same time increasing emotional intelligence and creativity. It may seem like you can't get any work done while you're asleep but the fact is that sleep enhances each and every function in your body, whether it's memory, immunity, appearance or functionality.

Among primates, only humans sleep flat on the ground or on the bed. This is because we have the highest proportion of REM sleep when the muscles go completely slack, at 20–25 per cent, as compared to primates, who have only 9 per cent and therefore are able to sleep arboreally (on trees). Scientists believe that it's this higher proportion of REM sleep that helped sharpen our minds and made us the leading species of our time.

To mine the innumerable benefits of deep slumber, it is important to ensure you're comfortable and also in a reasonably decent posture given that in the deepest stages, our body goes completely slack. Going to bed in the right posture has innumerable benefits, whether it's to sleep well or preserve spinal health. All of us have woken up to a sprain in the neck that takes days to fade away. Seema Sondhi, my yoga guru, would sleep with a tightly rolled hand towel placed under the thoracic region of her spine to open her chest and improve her standing posture. Indeed, it requires enormous discipline to utilize sleep to enhance the posture. But even if you don't want to make this time productive, ensuring you lie down correctly will, at the very least, improve the quality of your slumber.

1. Before you sleep, lie down for 10 minutes on your left side. In Ayurveda, this is called the *vamkukshi* position, considered the best to sleep as it is believed to aid digestion, detoxification and elimination. When you feel heavy or bloated, try to sleep on both sides and you'll find that the left side will help you feel lighter.

2. However, if you find that your mind is cluttered with overthinking, turn towards your right. Turning towards your right will open the left nostril. If you remember from the earlier chapters, one nostril is always more open, which governs our thoughts and bodily functions. The right nostril (pingala), ruled by the sun, is more active,

while the left nostril (ida), ruled by the moon, is more passive.

3. Keep your head supported with a thin pillow. It shouldn't be so high as to throw your neck out of alignment with the rest of your body.

4. Keep your legs slightly bent if you're sleeping on the side. Tuck a small cushion or pillow between your knees so that the hips don't go out of alignment and you're comfortable during the night.

5. If you sleep on your back, place a pillow under your knees so that the spine stays in a neutral position.

6. If you've been on your feet all day, slide a pillow under your feet to elevate them a little, so they de-bloat and feel rested by the morning.

7. If you sleep on your stomach, keep a pillow under the pelvis to keep your spine from dipping.

5

SLEEP AND CIRCADIAN RHYTHMS

In traditional sciences, living according to the circadian rhythms—going to bed and rising early—are key to a healthful life. In traditional medicine, be it Ayurveda or TCM, the body is governed by an internal clock. According to this ayurvedic clock, time is divided into four periods, each governed by one of the three doshas. The best time to sleep is before 10 p.m. because 6-10 p.m. belongs to the heavy kapha dosha, with slow and heavy elements of earth and water. If you notice, you may feel tired and sleepy during this time, an instinct that's usually ignored because it is too early to sleep. After 10 p.m., the fiery pitta dosha takes over, giving you a second wind. This boost of energy may be good for those who like to burn the midnight oil. For others (like me, who are most productive in the morning), it would do better to sleep before 10 p.m.

In the TCM organ clock, 24 hours are divided into 2-hour time slots, each corresponding to a particular organ. The period between 9 and 11 p.m. corresponds with the *san jiao* or the mysterious 'triple burner', which has no Western anatomical equal. Roughly translated, the san jiao is the meridian that influences the three 'burners' or 'energizers' in the body. The first is on the lungs and chest, the second between the diaphragm and navel and the third on the lower organs. Therefore, the san jiao corresponds with the overall rejuvenation and restoration of all the organs in the upper, middle and lower bodies. If you follow the TCM organ clock, then 9–11 p.m. is believed to be the right time to sleep as it triggers the internal repair and restoration of the body. Additionally, if you sleep during this period, you conserve energy required for internal bodily functions.

The Science of Sleep

Scientific studies show mixed results of synchronizing your sleep timings with natural circadian rhythms. But to understand sleep, we need to look at the two main stages of sleep NREM (non-rapid eye movement) and REM (rapid eye movement), which happen cyclically through the night. The former is a deep, dreamless sleep, which prevails in the first half of the night, while the latter is when you dream, that happens more during the second half on the night. Both stages of sleep are equally important—NREM helps regenerate the body, repair tissue and boost immunity, while REM sleep improves memory and learning.

Because REM sleep happens usually close to the morning, the ideal sleep hygiene would be to go to bed without setting an alarm, so that you're not jolted out of bed, thereby starving the mind of the REM sleep it deserves. To ensure you sleep without an alarm, you need to develop a disciplined daily routine. In an ideal world, you'd be asleep by 11 p.m., sleep for over 7 hours and wake up without an alarm. Even if you can't go to bed early, being a night owl (those who are predisposed to sleeping late), it is essential to cultivate a daily rhythm, so that the body can work with your sleeping habits instead of having to readjust on a daily basis.

It's not just the duration but consistency of sleep habits that counts. Irregular sleep schedules are associated with increased risk of health problems, such as obesity, high blood pressure and high cholesterol. You could make up the loss of sleep with an afternoon nap, but according to Ayurveda, napping is recommended more for older adults and in warm climates. Also, if you're an insomniac, it may prevent you from sleeping well at night.

Having said that, napping, when done right and for a short period, can help catch up on lost sleep. The ideal duration to feel refreshed is about 30 minutes. It's also essential to nap at the same time every day. If you can, do it sitting in an armchair so that the upper body stays elevated, because Ayurveda claims that lying down completely in the afternoon increases toxins in the bloodstream.

Ultimately, whether your sleep is monophasic (only at night) or biphasic (night and a nap in the day), a schedule is important so that the body knows when to begin the wind-down. This is why rituals are important, as they bring a sense of regularity in life.

The Sleep Mindset

If you've ever tried to give up smoking, you know that more than the actual process, it is the determination that helps you kick the habit. The same is with sleep. Today, we're addicted to our tablets and smartphones. Because there are a variety of options to keep us entertained the entire night, why would anyone ever want to sleep? To get a good night's rest, we have to *want* and prioritize it more than anything else. There's no podcast, series or conversation that cannot be postponed till the morning. Sleep has to be number one priority because it helps every function in our bodes—it's an anti-ageing pill, a memory enhancer, immunity booster all rolled into one. But nobody can spoon-feed you that motivation; you need to find it from within.

Easing out Stimulation

When we sleep well, we perform better the next day, our interpersonal relationships are better, we're inspired to work out, eat healthy and make the right choices. On the contrary, when we don't get enough sleep, we're not inspired to do anything at all. The first step of sleep hygiene then is to put away your phone, which will only happen when you are determined. Try replacing your smartphone or tablet with a book (especially one that is mildly academic/slow-paced). It may not be as stimulating as social media, but that is the whole point.

If you're an overthinker, it may be a good idea to write down a list of things to do the next day, lest you forget. In Ayurveda, this is especially recommended for the ambitious pitta type. Vata types do well with a warm oil foot massage that works to ground their flighty, anxious energy. Kapha types usually don't have a problem falling asleep—for them the problem is oversleeping. But whether it's journaling, meditation, massage or sound healing, the idea is to wind down and destress. The mind cannot run at a breakneck speed and then be expected to calm down and help you fall asleep.

Someone like me, who gets stimulated easily, prefers to either read a non-fiction/knowledge book or indulge in a sound bath before bed. Personally, I find that sometimes even reading on my phone is okay as long as I'm looking up information about beauty, health and wellness. For me, these are comforting areas of interest. For you, it could be language, astronomy or art history. If I get involved in an engaging conversation, I stay awake longer. So even if I'm on my phone, I avoid social media because I don't want to be faced with excitement, fear, revulsion, admiration or any other stimulating emotion right before bed.

The big worry is if we will be able to sleep at all. Often, the inability to fall asleep is what keeps us up all night. I remember reading an article about sleep management a while back on a particular night that I spent tossing and turning. It was almost 4 a.m. and I couldn't bear the thought of listening to the birdsong in the morning after a night I had laid awake. So I picked up my phone and looked up 'what can you do when you can't sleep all night'. Among the various tips the author had given, one line stood out so beautifully that I remember it to this day. A somnologist said something on the lines of 'ultimately you will go to sleep at some point, it may not come soon enough but it will come for sure'. I felt comforted by that and have worried a little bit less since then.

The paradox is that the moment we want to stay up is when we fall asleep the soonest. So if I'm wakeful in the middle of the night I like to do something, instead of just tossing in bed. I keep a heavy academic book, with difficult concepts, on my bedside table. It could also be an old, classic novel. Something heavy and verbose always makes me feel drowsy. But that's just me—we are all different and have different needs. Think about it like this—we feel the sleepiest when we're trying to stay awake. So instead of tossing and turning waiting for it to come, engage yourself in something boring. You could step out of the room for a few minutes, lie down and listen to a guided meditation, journal your thoughts. If you wake up in the middle of the night and aren't able to go to sleep, try one of these, or anything else that does not involve a screen.

Keep in mind that if sleep is a recurring problem, you may have a serious sleep disorder, for which you must contact a somnologist. There are about 80 different types of sleep disorders and if you have one, it's urgent you get the correct diagnosis. Alternative medicine protocols when combined with modern science work beautifully. Remember that sleep helps every other function in the body. So, if you suffer from a sleep disorder, the best self-care you can do is to visit the doctor and improve the quality of your life.

Think of sleep as nutrition. All of us have different needs when it comes to hours and timings of rest, just like we do in food. But making it a priority is essential for everyone. It's only when we sleep that we can enjoy the day. And it's only when we live the day to the fullest that we can sleep at night.

ACKNOWLEDGEMENTS

I want to thank the Penguin team—Gurveen Chadha my editor who's always been not only tolerant but also enthusiastic about my craziest schemes. Shreya Mukherjee for that last push that made this book happen. Akankgsha Sarmah for not following the brief and designing this breathtaking cover.

I'm grateful to my panel of experts for sharing their knowledge and patiently reading sections of my book. Dr Gunvant Yeola who deepened the information in my book with his vast knowledge on Ayurveda. Sudha Thimmaiyah my therapist, for reading through and giving insights on mental health. Deepika Mehta for guiding and refining the chapters on yoga. Dr Ipsita Chatterjee for her knowledge on ancient texts and their relevance in beauty and wellness. Rajni Ohri, for contributing traditional beauty recipes from her grandmother and along with massage practices.

My brother, my best friend Varun Rana (in bold caps) who edited the intros and introduced me to the world of prose.

Finally, this book wouldn't be complete without the unwavering support of Veena and Narendra, my parents, best friends and soulmates.

BIBLIOGRAPHY

Introduction

Besedovsky L and Lange T, Born J. 'Sleep and immune function'. *Pflugers Arch*. 463(1) (January 2012):121-37. doi: 10.1007/s00424-011-1044-0.

Kinouchi, K., Sassone-Corsi, P. 'Metabolic rivalry: circadian homeostasis and tumorigenesis'. *Nat Rev Cancer*. 20, (2020): 645–661. https://doi.org/10.1038/s41568-020-0291-9.

Nota, J.A., Coles, M.E. Duration and Timing of Sleep are Associated with Repetitive Negative Thinking. *Cogn Ther Res* 39, 253–261 (2015). https://doi.org/10.1007/s10608-014-9651-7.

Paddock, Catharine, Ph.D. 'REM Sleep Helps Solve Problems'. *MedicalNewsToday*. 9 June 2009.https://www.medicalnewstoday.com/articles/153189#1.

Serin Y, Acar. 'Effect of Circadian Rhythm on Metabolic Processes and the Regulation of Energy Balance'. *Ann Nutr Metab*. 74 (2019):322-330. doi: 10.1159/000500071.

Shin JE and Kim JK. 'How a Good Sleep Predicts Life Satisfaction: The Role of Zero-Sum Beliefs About Happiness'. *Front Psychol*. 28;9 (August 2018):1589. doi: 10.3389/fpsyg.2018.01589.

Nurture

FACE MASSAGE— Cho, Yoon Soo, et al. 'The effect of burn rehabilitation massage therapy on hypertrophic scar after burn: A randomized controlled trial'. *Burns*. Volume 40, Issue 8 (2014):1513-1520. https://www.sciencedirect.com/science/article/pii/S0305417914000655.

BODY MASSAGE—Agarwal, Kailash and Gupta, A & Pushkarna, R & Bhargava, Krishnakant & Faridi, Mma & Prabhu, M. 'Effects of massage & use of oil on growth, blood flow & sleep pattern in infants'. *The Indian journal of medical research*. 112. (2010): 212-7.

BODY MASSAGE—Vanitha, N., Prof. Annie Annal, M. and Dr. Renuka K. 'An experimental study to evaluate the effectiveness of application of almond oil massage on breast feeding among postnatal mothers undergone lscs at MGMCRI Puducherry'. *Internation Journal of Current Research*.http://www.journalcra.com/article/experimental-study-evaluate-effectiveness-application-almond-oil-massage-breast-feeding.

BODY MASSAGE—Nethravathi V and Vijaitha V. 'Effectiveness of Clove oil massage on Lower Back Pain among Post Natal Mothers at Selected Hospitals, Bangalore'. *Asian J. Nur. Edu. and Research* 5(4) (October- December 2015): 467-470. https://ajner.com/AbstractView.aspx?PID=2015-5-4-5.

FACE MASSAGE—H. Nishimura, I. et al. 'Amano Analysis of morphological changes after facial massage by a novel approach using three-dimensional computed tomography'. *Skin Research & Technology*, Volume 23, issue 3 (22 November 2016). https://doi.org/10.1111/srt.12345.

FACE MASSAGE—Caberlotto E, et al. 'Effects of a skin-massaging device on the ex-vivo expression of human dermis proteins and in-vivo facial wrinkles'. *PLoS One*. 1;12(3) (March 2017):e0172624. doi: 10.1371/journal.pone.0172624.

FACE MASSAGE—Vinacci, John. 'Human Physiology and Muscle Anatomy for Massage Therapists'. https://s3.amazonaws.com/EliteCME_WebSite_2013/f/pdf/MIL04HPI14.pdf.

FACE MASSAGE—Chamberlain, Gail J. 'Cyriax's Friction Massage: A Review'. *The Journal of Orthopaedic and Sports Physical Therapy*. https://www.jospt.org/doi/pdf/10.2519/jospt.1982.4.1.16.

FOOT MASSAGE— Sarmah, Jyoti Manab, et al. 'A Conceptual Study on Dristiprasadana of Padabhyagana'. *International Ayurvedic Medical Journal*. http://www.iamj.in/posts/2019/images/upload/1572_1575.pdf.

FOOT MASSAGE—Joshi, Nitesh and Ujwale, Ramesh. 'A CLINICAL STUDY OF THE EFFECT OF TILA TAILA PADABHYANGA ON EYE STRAIN'. *International Journal of Research in Ayurveda & Pharmacy*. 7. (2016):29-35. 10.7897/2277-4343.07250.

HEAD MASSAGE—Kim IH, et al. 'The effect of a scalp massage on stress hormone, blood pressure, and heart rate of healthy female'. *J Phys Ther Sci*. 28(10) (October 2016):2703-2707. doi: 10.1589/jpts.28.2703.

HEAD MASSAGE—Koyama T, et al. 'Standardized Scalp Massage Results in Increased Hair Thickness by Inducing Stretching Forces to Dermal Papilla Cells in the Subcutaneous Tissue'. *Eplasty*. 25;16 (January 2016):e8. PMID: 26904154.

HEAD MASSAGE—Murota M, et al. 'Physical and Psychological Effects of Head Treatment in the Supine Position Using Specialized Ayurveda-Based Techniques'. *J Altern Complement Med*. 22(7) (July 2016):526-32. doi: 10.1089/acm.2015.0388.

HEAL STUDY— Miquel-Kergoat, Sophie, et al. 'Effects of chewing on appetite, food intake and gut hormones: A systematic review and meta-analysis'. *Physiology & Behavior*. Volume 151 (2015):88-96. https://www.sciencedirect.com/science/article/pii/S0031938415300317.

HEAL STUDY—American Heart Association. 'Dog ownership associated with longer life, especially among heart attack and stroke survivors'. *ScienceDaily*. www.sciencedaily.com/releases/2019/10/191008083121.htm.

HEAL STUDY— Beaulieu, Johnhttp. 'BioSonics, Stress Science, and Nitric Oxide Literature Review'. http//www.biosonics.com/uploads2011/BioSonicsStressScienceandNO.pdf.

HEAL STUDY—The Healthline Editorial Team. 'Having Trouble Sleeping? Try a Hot Bath Before Bed'. Healthline. (25 July 2019). https://www.healthline.com/health-news/having-trouble-sleeping-try-a-hot-bath-before-bed.

Luo Y, Chen X, Qi S, You X and Huang X. 'Well-being and Anticipation for Future Positive Events: Evidences from an fMRI Study'. *Front Psychol*. 9;8 (2018):2199. doi: 10.3389/fpsyg.2017.02199.

PRANAYAMA—Ankad RB, et al. 'Effect of short-term pranayama and meditation on cardiovascular functions in healthy individuals'. *Heart Views*. 12(2) (April 2011):58-62. doi: 10.4103/1995-705X.86016.

NABHI PURAN—Chien Y. W. 'Long-term controlled navel administration of testosterone'. *Journal of pharmaceutical sciences*, *73*(8) (1984): 1064–1067. https://doi.org/10.1002/jps.2600730811.

NABHI PURAN—DiPatrizio NV. 'Endocannabinoids in the Gut'. *Cannabis Cannabinoid Res*. 1(1) (February 2016):67-77. doi: 10.1089/can.2016.0001.

NABHI PURAN— Kalekar, Dr Vishnupriya. 'A New Approach in Management of Amenorrhoea wsr to Mrutthika Basti Chikitsa and in Katigraha wsr to Vacuum Therapy: A Case Study'. *Ayurved Darpan Journal of Indian Medicine*. http://www.ayurveddarpan.com/AyurVed/journal/99_1.pdf.

NABHI PURAN—Liu, Zhe, et al. 'Acupoint herbal patching at Shenque (CV8) as an adjunctive therapy for acute diarrhea in children: A systematic review and meta-analysis'. *European Journal of Integrative Medicine*. Volume 10 (2017): 25-37. https://www.sciencedirect.com/science/article/pii/S1876382017300094.

UBTAN—Biswas, Rajarshi et al. 'Evaluation of Ubtan- A Traditional Indian Skin Care Formulation'. *Journal of Ethnopharmacology*. (2016). 192. 10.1016/j.jep.2016.07.034.

UDVARTHANA—Verma, Jatinder et al. 'Udvartana (Ayurveda Powder Massage): A Review Article'. (2019). https://www.researchgate.net/publication/333866630_Udvartana_Ayurveda_Powder_Massage_A_Review_Article#:~:text=It%20is%20a%20simple%20and,vitiated%20Kapha%20and%20Meda)%20properties.

Heal

FOOD HABITS—Miquel-Kergoat, Sophie, et al. 'Effects of chewing on appetite, food intake and gut hormones: A systematic review and meta-analysis'. *Physiology & Behavior* Volume 151 (2015):88-96. https://www.sciencedirect.com/science/article/pii/S0031938415300317.

JOURNALLING—Koopman C, et al. 'The effects of expressive writing on pain, depression and post traumatic stress disorder symptoms in survivors of intimate partner violence'. *Health Psychol.* 10(2)(March 2005):211-21. doi: 10.1177/1359105305049769.

JOURNALLING—Mugerwa S, Holden JD. 'Writing therapy: a new tool for general practice?' *Br J Gen Pract.* 62(605) (December 2012):661-3. doi: 10.3399/bjgp12X659457.

JOURNALLING—Pennebaker JW. 'Traumatic experience and psychosomatic disease: Exploring the roles of behavioural inhibition, obsession, and confiding'. *Can Psychol.* 1985;26:82–95.

JOURNALLING—Petrie, K. J., et al. 'Effect of written emotional expression on immune function in patients with human immunodeficiency virus infection: a randomized trial'. *Psychosomatic medicine*, 66(2), (2004): 272–275. https://doi.org/10.1097/01.psy.0000116782.49850.d3.

SOUND HEALING—Beutel ME, et al. 'Noise Annoyance Is Associated with Depression and Anxiety in the General Population-The Contribution of Aircraft Noise'. *PLoS One.*11(5) (19 May 2016):e0155357. doi: 10.1371/journal.pone.0155357.

SOUND HEALING—Chaieb L, Wilpert, et al. 'Auditory beat stimulation and its effects on cognition and mood States'. *Front Psychiatry.* 6:70 (12 May 2015). doi: 10.3389/fpsyt.2015.00070.

SOUND HEALING— Bardekar, A.A. and Gurjar, Ajay.A. 'Empirical Study of Indian Classical Ragas Structure and its Emotional Influence on Human Body For Music Therapy'. *Journal of Management Engineering and Information Technology.* (August 2016). http://www.jmeit.com/JMEIT_Vol_3_Issue_4_Aug_2016/JMEIT0304001.pdf

SOUND HEALING—Jenkins JS. 'The Mozart effect'. *J R Soc Med.*94(4) (April 2001):170-2. doi: 10.1177/014107680109400404.

SOUND HEALING—Kučikienė D and Praninskienė R. 'The impact of music on the bioelectrical oscillations of the brain'. *Acta Med Litu.* 25(2) (2018):101-106. doi: 10.6001/actamedica.v25i2.3763.

SOUND HEALING—Kumar, Kamakhya. 'Effect of Learning Music as a Practice of Nada Yoga on EEG Alpha and General Well Being'. *Yoga Mimamsa.* 43 (2011): 215-20.

SOUND HEALING—Sanivarapu SL. 'India's rich musical heritage has a lot to offer to modern psychiatry'. *Indian J Psychiatry.* 57(2) (April-June- 2015):210-3. doi: 10.4103/0019-5545.158201. PMID: 26124532; PMCID: PMC4462795.

SOUND HEALING—Winkelman M. 'Complementary therapy for addiction: "drumming out drugs"'. *Am J Public Health.* 93(4) (April 2003):647-51. doi: 10.2105/ajph.93.4.647.

Rest

BELLY BREATHING—Ma X, et al. 'The Effect of Diaphragmatic Breathing on Attention, Negative Affect and Stress in Healthy Adults'. *Front Psychol.* 8:874 (6 June 2017). doi: 10.3389/fpsyg.2017.00874.

BRAHMARI— Kuppusamy M, et al. 'Effects of *Bhramari Pranayama* on health - A systematic review'. *J Tradit Complement Med.* 8(1) (18 March 2017):11-16. doi: 10.1016/j.jtcme.2017.02.003.

BREATHE DEEPLY— Joseph, Chacko N., et al. 'Slow Breathing Improves Arterial Baroreflex Sensitivity and Decreases Blood Pressure in Essential Hypertension'. *Hypertension* V 46, N 4(2005): 714-718. https://www.ahajournals.org/doi/abs/10.1161/01.HYP.0000179581.68566.7d.

BREATHE DEEPLY— Saoji AA, et al. 'Effects of yogic breath regulation: A narrative review of scientific evidence'.

Ayurveda Integr Med. 10(1)(2019):50-58. doi: 10.1016/j. jaim.2017.07.008.

BREATHE DEEPLY—Yackle, Kevin, et al. 'Breathing control center neurons that promote arousal in mice'. Science. V 355, number 6332 (2017): 1411-1415. doi: 10.1126/science. aai7984.

PREPARING FOR REST—West, Kathleen E., et al. 'Blue light from light-emitting diodes elicits a dose-dependent suppression of melatonin in humans'. *Journal of Applied Physiology*. volume 110, issue 3 (1 March 2011). https://doi. org/10.1152/japplphysiol.01413.2009.

PHYSIOLOGICAL SIGHS—Elke Vlemincx, et al. 'A sigh of relief or a sigh to relieve: The psychological and physio.logical relief effect of deep breaths'. *Physiology & Behavior*, Volume 165(2016): 127-135, https://www.sciencedirect.com/science/ article/pii/S0031938416305121.

SLEEP AND CIRCADIAN RHYTHM—*Science Direct*. https:// www.sciencedirect.com/topics/medicine-and-dentistry/triple- energizer.

SLEEP AND CIRCADIAN RHYTHM—Chaput JP, et al. 'Sleeping hours: what is the ideal number and how does age impact this?' *Nat Sci Sleep*.10 (27 November 2018):421-430. doi: 10.2147/NSS.S163071.

SLEEP AND CIRCADIAN RHYTHM—Chuangshi Wang, et al. 'Association of bedtime with mortality and major cardiovascular events: an analysis of 112,198 individuals from 21 countries in the PURE study'. *Sleep Medicine*. Volume 80 (2021): 265-272. https://doi.org/10.1016/j.sleep.2021. 01.057.

SLEEP AND CIRCADIAN RHYTHM— Knutson, Kristen L. and von Schantz, Malcolm. 'Associations between chronotype, morbidity and mortality in the UK Biobank cohort'.

Chronobiology International 35:8 (2018): 1045-1053, DOI: 10.1080/07420528.2018.1454458.

SLEEP AND CIRCADIAN RHYTHM— Huang, Tianyi, et al. 'Cross-sectional and Prospective Associations of Actigraphy-Assessed Sleep Regularity With Metabolic Abnormalities: The Multi-Ethnic Study of Atherosclerosis'. *Diabetes Care* 42 (8)(1 August 2019): 1422–1429. https://doi.org/10.2337/dc19-0596.

SLEEP BEVERAGES— Friedman M. 'Analysis, Nutrition, and Health Benefits of Tryptophan'. *Tryptophan Res.* (26 September 2018). doi: 10.1177/1178646918802282.

SLEEP BEVERAGES—Kim S, et al. 'GABA and l-theanine mixture decreases sleep latency and improves NREM sleep'. *Pharm Biol.* 57(1) December 2019):65-73. doi: 10.1080/13880209.2018.1557698.

SLEEP BEVERAGES—Langade, Deepak, et al. 'Clinical evaluation of the pharmacological impact of ashwagandha root extract on sleep in healthy volunteers and insomnia patients: A double-blind, randomized, parallel-group, placebo-controlled study'. *Journal of Ethnopharmacology*, Volume 264, 2021.

SLEEP BEVERAGES—Nathan, P. et al. 'The neuropharmacology of L-theanine(N-ethyl-L-glutamine): a possible neuroprotective and cognitive enhancing agent;. *Journal of herbal pharmacotherapy*, 6(2) (2006). 21–30.

SLEEP BEVERAGES—Toolika E, et al. 'A comparative clinical study on the effect of Tagara (Valeriana wallichii DC.) and Jatamansi (Nardostachys jatamansi DC.) in the management of Anidra (primary insomnia)'. *Ayu.* 36(1) (January-March 2015):46-9. doi: 10.4103/0974-8520.169008.

Books for Moon

Flaws, Bob. *Curing Fibromyalgia Naturally With Chinese Medicine.* (Blue Poppy, 2000).

McBride, Shaman Melodie. *Going Towards the Nature Is Going Towards the Health.* (US: Xlibris, 2012).

Nishi, Katsuzo. *The Nishi System of Health Engineering.* (US: Kessinger Publishing, 2010).

Pitchford, Paul. *Healing with Whole Foods: Asian Traditions and Modern Nutrition.* (US: North Atlantic Books, 2002).

Saraswati, Swami Satyananda. *Asana Pranayama Mudra Bandha.* (Munger: Bihar School of Yoga, 2008).

Thompson, Richard L. *Vedic Cosmography and Astronomy.* (Motilal Banarsidass Publishers, 2003).

ABOUT THE EXPERTS

Dr Gunvant Yeola, MD, PhD (Kayachikitsa) is an Ayurveda physician, principal, professor and head of Kayachikitsa department at Dr D.Y. Patil College of Ayurved and Research Centre, Pune. He is also consultant at Vedansh Ayurved Clinic and Tanman Ayurvedic Research Centre, Pune. He is regularly invited for lectures and consultations in Portugal, the Netherlands, USA and Brazil, and is an established name in the world of Ayurveda.

Deepika Mehta is one of India's most prominent ashtanga yoga teachers. A level-two authorized teacher from KPJAYI, her experience of more than two decades has made her a leading figure in the world of fitness. Deepika began practising yoga to heal from a back injury. Her teachings stem from a place of healing, and her trademark style combines dance with traditional yoga, making ashtanga more accessible for all.

Sudha Thimmaiah Sudha is a senior therapist with Anna Chandy & Associates, Bengaluru. An internationally certified counsellor, she comes with decades of experience in helping clients across age groups deal with addiction, complex relationships, work–life balance, depression and anxiety. Her personal experience of breaking through her own systemic hierarchical patterns of thinking and beliefs has empowered her to work with clients on their need for individual identity within their family systems and in the larger context of expectations of society.

Lovneet Batra is a sports nutritionist who has counselled the Indian boxing, gymnastics, cycling and archery teams during the Commonwealth Games. She is a consultant for the Fortis Group of Hospitals and a visiting faculty at IHM Pusa, New Delhi, in the department of New Product Development and Sports Nutrition. She is the founder of Nutrition by Lovneet and author of the book *Fifty Desi Super Drinks*.

Dr Ipsita Chatterjee has a master's degree in Ayurvedic Rasashastra and Bhaishaiya Kalpana (a branch dealing with Ayurvedic pharmaceutics

and cosmetics). She is an Ayurvedic scientist who has worked with the leading names in the Indian Ayurvedic industry. She has over a decade's experience in branded luxury Ayurveda and retail, and also has consulted with patients on wellness, diet and lifestyle.

Rajni Ohri is the founder of the award-winning Ayurvedic brand Ohria Ayurveda. She has also devised a bespoke Ageless Face Yoga Programme and personalized massage rituals. She has done advanced courses with face yoga pioneers such as Koko Hayashi from Japan and Vasiliki Pissa from Greece. She has also learnt advanced aromatherapy from Shirley Price in London.

· SUN ·

RITUAL

Daily Practices for

WELLNESS, BEAUTY

& BLISS

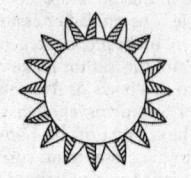

VASUDHA RAI

EBURY
PRESS

An imprint of Penguin Random House

EBURY PRESS

USA | Canada | UK | Ireland | Australia
New Zealand | India | South Africa | China

Ebury Press is part of the Penguin Random House group of companies
whose addresses can be found at global.penguinrandomhouse.com

Published by Penguin Random House India Pvt. Ltd
4th Floor, Capital Tower 1, MG Road,
Gurugram 122 002, Haryana, India

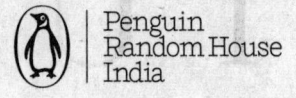

Penguin
Random House
India

First published in Ebury Press by Penguin Random House India 2022

ISBN 9780143452935

Typeset in Adobe Garamond Pro by Manipal Technologies Limited, Manipal
Printed at Replika Press Pvt. Ltd, India

www.penguin.co.in

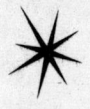

For Krishna Reya, my badmash, my lucky charm

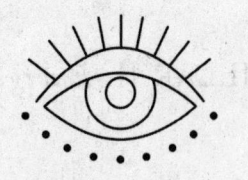

CONTENTS

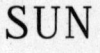 

✳

~~~~~ PILLAR II: *Energize* ~~~~~

✳

~~~~~ PILLAR II: *Focus* ~~~~~

INTRODUCTION

An Ode to the Day

*The dawn splits open the shell of darkness, illuminating
the heavens with golden light. The Sun has risen. In those
early moments, the world is still quiet, its senses awakening
slowly with the brightening sky. And just as slowly, all
our senses—smell, taste, touch, sound, and sight—are
heightened, brought back to life by the Sun's gilded rays.
The atmosphere transforms with luminosity, warmth,
and lightness, washing away the sediments of the just-
departed darkness.*

*The masculine Sun with its expansive power that moves
outwards, far and wide. This golden orb pushes us to
mimic its blinding light. The expansive energy of El Sol
controls the physical world, its awake mind and conscious
actions. In all its power and potency, the Sun brings your
attention to the tangible present, maximizing the here and
now. While Time runs on like sand through your fingers,
the Sun reminds us, strong warriors all, to never stop—to
embrace our fiery side, to reach out with both hands and to
grab the moment.*

*Solar energy expands and stretches matter, it's warmth
also opens our hearts. It tells us not to be afraid of the fire
because we are made up of the light that we seek. Look at
the sun so hot and powerful but it sets itself alight from the
very core. Only then can it share its generous warmth and
energises us with its benevolent light.*

*And as it sets, the Sun leaves us with the promise of
another day. Even if things aren't done, there's always
tomorrow. A symbol of permanence, the Sun moves reliably
from East to West. Because of it, everything is cyclical, not
just the phases of the Night and Day. So fear not if there's
still much to be said and done. You too will get another
chance when the majestic Sun rises again.*

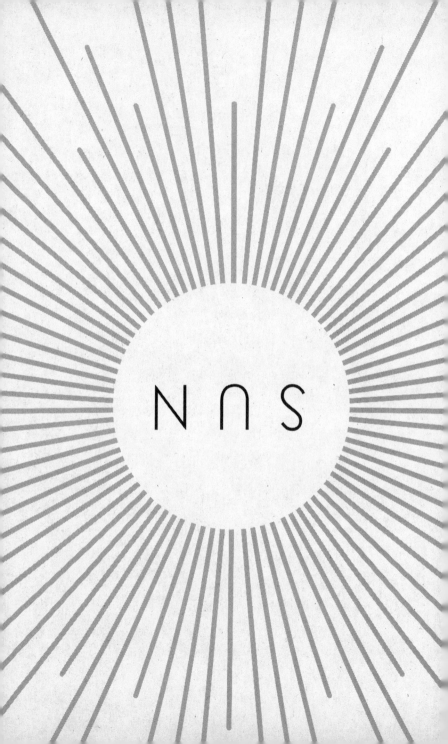

It's about 3,33,000 times the size of our planet. Were it hollow, a million earths would fit inside the sun. It accounts for more than 99 per cent of the mass in our solar system and coverts about 400 million tonnes of matter into energy every second. It's our primary source of nourishment, giving us food and energy. It regulates our metabolism, boosts the mood and also regulates sleep/wake cycles in most organisms. It's no surprise then that for us humans, the sun is a symbol of growth, renewal and hope. Because it wields such an enormous influence on our health and well-being, it enjoys an exalted status, and is seen as a divine presence in many cultures.

In past civilizations, the sun has inspired innumerable tales of magnificence. The Vedas accurately credit it as being the harbinger of life, creating all that exists on the physical plane. In keeping with this worshipped Ra, the sun god belief, the Vedic civilization was centred on the worship of the sun and of fire. In the Japanese Shinto system, essentially worship of nature, the position of the sun goddess Amaterasu was elevated over other deities. The Aztecs called themselves people of the sun, the Egyptians worshipped Ra, the sun god, while the Romans adopted the image of the sun, *sol invictus* (the invincible sun), to represent their solar deity.

In the last century, we've gone beyond mythological references and have understood how the cyclical patterns

of the sun impact human body and mind. Circadian rhythms govern the functioning of every living being, from microorganisms to humans. We know now that living according to these rhythms is the ultimate investment in health. When we live in harmony with the natural cycles of day and night, it benefits cognitive function, metabolism and physical fitness. Even something as minute as our cell cycle, in which cells replicate their DNA and subsequently divide, is controlled by the circadian clock. Therefore, following the sun's lead is as important as the right diet and exercise.

There is some evidence to show that those who wake up around sunrise are more proactive and productive. The connection between productivity and early waking time is clear even in those who prefer to sleep in. When late risers reprogrammed their routines to sleep and wake up earlier, they found an improvement in mental health and performance. But even if you're not a morning person, you can reap the benefits of the sun by exposing yourself to bouts of sunshine. It has been found that exposure to sunlight helps lower blood pressure, boost levels of serotonin in the brain and even improve digestion and gut health.

The moment sunlight hits the photoreceptors in the retina, it sends a signal to the brain, increasing alertness in humans. In ideal conditions, this would mean that the day brings with it energy and focus to get though the tasks on our to-do lists. However, over the past few decades, we have completely disconnected with circadian rhythms. Earlier, the lack of electricity meant that we were forced to retire to bed after sunset. But today, though technology has made

everything more convenient, it has made us disconnect with the natural rhythms. It's normal now to feel sleepy in the day and energized at night.

Admittedly, not everyone should wake up with the first rays of dawn, and certainly not at the cost of sleep. However, reversing the circadian clock over the long term is like playing Russian roulette with health. To live well, we must learn to harness the powers of daylight and work with the body's natural rhythms. For that, three elemental daytime processes need to be enhanced:

1. Purify—to begin on a clean state.
2. Energize—to propel into action.
3. Focus—to streamline your thoughts.

Think of these as the three pillars of the sun. Neither exists in isolation; each is inextricably linked with the other. Most importantly, with these pillars, we aren't working against the natural tendencies, but harmonizing with them.

The process of purification is essential to eliminate sediments of the night, clear one's mental fog and refresh oneself from the inside out. Gut-clearing a.m. elixirs, energizing showers, cleansing *kriyas*, fasts and detoxes (all part of the morning cleanse) have exponential benefits. Something as simple as the temperature of your bath water could either sap or boost your energy. Your morning drink can, in fact, set the tone for the day. The practice of fasting has been revived around the world for its ability to reset body and mind. Even a quick and effortless a.m. ritual like oiling the nostrils helps prevent infections and builds immunity.

 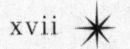

Energy, the second pillar of the sun, is known as *virya*, or bravery, when translated to Sanskrit or Pali language. Virya is commonly used in Buddhism to denote diligence, effort or eagerness, all of which depend upon us feeling energized. Within the realm of yoga, the right nostril, which holds the *surya nadi*, has great significance, especially when it comes to energy. To digress briefly, nadis are etheric nerves, or meridians, as they're called in Traditional Chinese Medicine (TCM). The three main nadis in the body are the surya nadi in the right nostril, *chandra nadi* in the left nostril and the *shushumna*, which runs down the centre of our spine. The surya nadi is responsible for regulating the more active functions of the body, such as physical work or digestion. Also called *pingala*, this nadi generates heat and provides the vigour to go out and achieve our goals. It mirrors the energy of the sun and daytime, where the emphasis is on work, energy, focus and clarity. This section will outline not just how to activate the pingala, but also exercise and breath work, mid-day stretches, nutrition and refreshing teas.

While energy gives you the push towards action, it can be scattered without focus. What does it mean to have a centre of attention? I learnt the true meaning of this at a vipassana retreat a few years back. While practising breath meditation, over the course of a few days, we were asked to make the area of focus smaller each day until we were asked to concentrate on just the sensation of breath on the line of the upper lip. We were explained that the smaller the area of focus, the sharper the brain develops, with practice. Call it attention to detail if you will. This section reveals the practices of *trataka*, *mudra*,

mantra, meditation and prayer, which work to control and refine the mind.

Each of these pillars has myriad interpretations, but just like millennial routines, modern rituals too are bespoke. Even though every one of us has a predictable rhythm, it can still greatly vary from one to the other. I'm most productive in the morning but my friend sits down to work after dinner. Health is a priority for both of us, but we look for different elements to enrich our lives.

A quarter of a century earlier, we had to plan every aspect of our lives. The lack of smartphones that meant meetings were planned in advance and tickets booked well in time. But today, we have the power in our hands. We can change plans with a text and block tickets with the click of a button. Lifestyles are now more whimsical than ever before.

Therefore, while it is undeniably beneficial to harness these energies during the hours of sunshine, they can be beneficial in the night too. If you're demotivated, lethargic or prone to procrastination, you may require this energy irrespective of the time of the day. It is sometimes required for us to be focused at night and relaxed during the day. Therefore, rituals can be chosen depending not just on the time but also the requirement. The ideal time to practise the rituals outlined in this part of the book is obviously during daylight hours. However, if you're a night owl, you may want to utilize some of these practices after dark to increase your energy, focus and productivity.

Ultimately, the energy of the sun is driven by hope. This simple word has a modern interpretation—manifestation—a word so overused that it has almost lost its magic. I prefer

to hope, which gives us the energy to do things instead of actively manifesting, which drains energy. Being hopeful is looking at each morning as another opportunity, one more chance for a do-over. Perhaps it'll be better than yesterday or maybe not. But either way, when the sun sets, even if things didn't go according to plan, we can expect them to be better tomorrow, when the day dawns afresh.

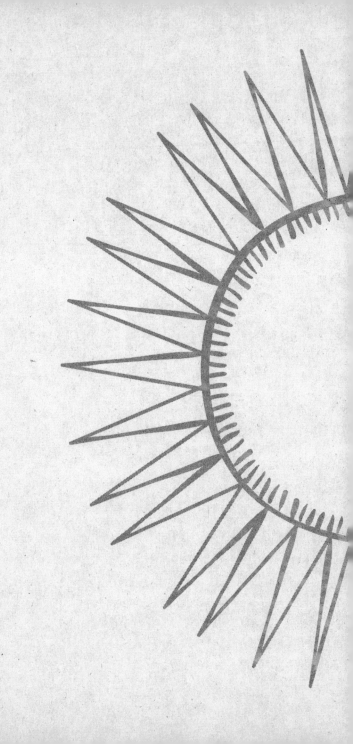

PILLAR I

✳

Purify

> If you are irritated by every rub, how will your mirror be polished?
>
> —Rumi

Every new project begins on a clean slate, because we can't paint on a dirty canvas. We think of cleansing—an essential component of everyday living—only in its outermost manifestation, such as, a daily bath or brushing our teeth. But even the simple act of bathing goes beyond physical cleanliness as it's also a reflection of how we feel in our mind. Along with these obvious practices, cleansing also includes deeper levels of purification—we can cleanse with our breath, a meditative practice or a deep detox that requires rigour and discipline.

The most intensive cleanse I ever had was at a twenty-one-day panchakarma retreat. It required enemas, purgation and sweating, along with spartan meals. It was hard, but for me, it was worth it. As someone who has been consistently on painkillers and synthetic hormones, I found it beneficial to remove (what felt like) waste circulating in my body. After twenty-one days, every part of my body—from my fingernails to the roof of my mouth—felt smooth and renewed. It may not work for many people because of the time and discipline

involved, but it worked for me. Panchakarma taught me the importance of internal cleansing. It doesn't have to be as intense, but small purification practices on the daily, such as rituals like *neti* or *nasya*, or purifying herbal teas, can build health in tiny instalments.

If you think about it, the concept of *saucha*, which is cleanliness or hygiene, goes beyond the external body and into the realm of purity of our internal organs, our surroundings, speech, senses and mind. Therefore, you can choose from a multitude of methods to purify at every level. Some such as breathwork, are indulgent and comforting, but others, like panchakarma, can be fairly challenging. Such a high degree of cleanliness in every aspect may seem a like a tall order, therefore, one must only do what can be continued comfortably. Even though there are many rituals outlined in the following chapters, it's better to choose no more than one or two and then slowly build up, if required.

After a brief romance with microbes, the COVID-19 masterclass in 2020 reminded us that personal hygiene can save lives. Indeed, cleansing is especially relevant in these times, when pollution is at an all-time high.

But hygiene isn't just a sterile space with rubber gloves and steel instruments. Think of a bath, which can be refreshing or indulgent, but therapeutic either way. A cold shower in the morning awakens the mind, whereas warm baths in the evening are so relaxing that they may reduce the risk of cardiovascular disease in the elderly. Weirdly enough, there is some evidence to show that washing hands makes us feel optimistic after failing at a task. Perhaps just

the act of washing something makes us ready to renew our efforts.

Ayurveda outlines detailed practices that involve cleansing and oiling the face and body. At first, you may not want to overburden yourself with additional rituals, especially when you're rushed for time. However, these practices aren't just for the purpose of removing grime, but to open the sense organs, balance hormones and help keep you strong as you grow older. Over time, as you practise these kriyas, you'll find great solace in breath without obstruction, sight without strain and sound without congestion.

While it is perfectly okay to stick to a single activity, for best results, purity must be seen as a synchronized concept for refined, elevated living: the mind, body and our environment are all interdependent. We cannot live with a clean body and a chaotic mind, or a purified mind with cluttered surroundings. Each aspect of purity affects the other. To achieve harmony between body, mind and surroundings, we need synchronistic action. Research has found that the inhabitants of homes teeming with clutter and unfinished projects had greater levels of stress and fatigue. Even within in the realm of decluttering, we can find magic with energy clearing practises such as using *loban*, incense, resins and sea salt, which make a home feel more purified.

But other than clearing just the surroundings, we also need to process and flush out thoughts that erode our peace of mind. While hygiene is the benchmark for health and wellness, purity also means refined thoughts. With the advent of social media, we're bombarded every minute with opinions, news, advice and microaggression via our smartphones. Viewed

first thing in the morning, this information overload—also known as infobesity—negatively impacts consciousness and clouds the mind. Studies have proved that social media increases anxiety, challenges cognitive capacity, destroys self-confidence and also causes untidiness. It has been suggested that just clicking back and forth between your smartphone and an important project can reduce productivity by up to 40 per cent.

To be able to use modern technology with control, it is essential to cultivate clarity of thought or mental hygiene. In the Zen tradition, it is said that there is actually no difference between the mundane mind and the Buddha mind. Everyone is born with the same faculties; the difference is that the Buddha mind is completely pure and free of obstruction. There are many ways to clear the mind, ranging from physical practices to everyday habits. It is important to understand that every element of purification will lead to a higher rung of clarity, thereby increasing productivity.

In these chapters, we will begin from the time of waking up and go through purification processes such as cleansing kriyas, baths, mantras, detoxes and fasting. While most of the rituals in this section are physical, they work to bestow a feeling of lightness, energy and enhanced mental acuity. Think of this as the bottom of the pyramid of the sun. A thorough purification of the body, mind and senses is elementary, before you graduate towards subtler practices of breath and meditation.

1

WAKING UP WITH CLARITY

Your mind is at its purest when you wake up. Marcel Proust called it the sleep of lead, that heavy mental state when sleep extends into consciousness upon waking up. In the first few moments, it's almost like the brain has forgotten what happened the night before. Awakening from the slow delta waves of deep sleep, the brain is in the alpha stage, considered to be the gateway to the subconscious. During this stage of purity, between sleep and wakefulness, it is the worst idea to reach for your phone. After all, you don't want the chatter from your inbox to be imprinted into your mind.

We know that the usage of smartphones increases anxiety, but researchers have also found clear links between smartphone usage and increased levels of stress, depression and low self-esteem. However, you don't need a study to tell you how your phone makes you feel. Conversely, abstaining from smartphone use in the bedroom leads to increased levels of happiness, but you don't need a study to know this either. There is nothing so urgent that it cannot wait for an hour after waking up. At the very least, make the first half an

hour about connecting with your breath, offering gratitude, affirming or just being in the moment—all activities which positively impact the subconscious mind.

Sleep has the ability to temporarily dissolve trauma, especially in the first few moments upon waking up, when you are suspended between the two worlds of dream and reality. For those couple of seconds, there seems to be no reason to stress, unless of course you pick up your phone. The way we wake up has the ability to refine the mind and keep it at ease. Whether it's choosing the right alarm or harmonious mental and physical activities, keep your mornings calm and centred for a clear, fruitful day.

1. Choose the Right Alarm

In an ideal world, we would wake up without an alarm. When it rings in the morning, the sound of an alarm usually yanks you out of a dream. This dreamlike state is the REM phase of sleep, which nourishes the mind, balances emotions and boosts creativity. Therefore, when an alarm goes off, it shaves time off your REM sleep, which is crucial for rejuvenating the mind. Following a disciplined daily routine will help you wake up naturally, even before the alarm goes off. But for most of us, alarms provide the assurance that we will wake up and make it to work on time.

Until you train your body clock to wake up naturally, choosing the right alarm will wake you up gently, without shocking the mind. Interestingly, it was found that waking up to a melodious alarm can help reduce sleep inertia (that disoriented feeling when you wake up) as compared to a

harsh beep. To be exact, researchers called it music that you can hum to, which, in a way, warms up your mind, just like you warm up your body before exercise.

2. Skip the Snooze Button

The snooze button is the usual escape, which causes a fluctuation in energy when you go from wakefulness to sleep. So, the second step (after choosing the right alarm) is to try to never snooze. Once you're awake with an alarm, stay in that wakeful state. Attempting to sleep again will leave you in an in-between state where you're neither awake nor asleep. The problem is that first you disturb your REM sleep with an alarm, then you go to sleep and are woken again in the middle of this second nap with the snooze button. By habitually pressing snooze, you will swing between wakefulness and deep sleep, which will lead you to feel lazy all day.

According to Ayurveda, the hours between 6 and 10 a.m. are the kapha part of the day. During this time, the environment embodies kapha qualities—heavy, earthy, dense and dull. Another reason yogis recommend waking up before sunrise is because it is the vata time of the day. The environment then embodies the ethereal qualities of lightness, air and ether, which make up the vata dosha.

3. Attune the Mind

My grandfather used to say that it is a miracle to wake up, be alive and well to see another day. Remind yourself of this stroke of luck when you open your eyes. My father looks at his palms first thing in the morning. He says that he does this because he is grateful to have hands that have worked and shaped his life. Ayurvedic vaidyas claim that this gesture helps cap the ego and helps show gratitude to the universe. It's a simple ritual that's better than reaching out for the phone. Your subconscious mind is most active within 20 minutes of waking up. It is prudent then to utilize this time doing activities that make you want to positively impact your subconscious mind.

The first few minutes can be spent reconnecting with your breath, meditating or making an affirmation. I find that affirmations work beautifully when you're insecure about the day. One of my favourite affirmations is 'Every day in every way I get better and better.' You could also begin the day with gratitude, thinking about three things that you are thankful for this morning. Or you could just lie in bed and take 10-25 deep breaths to centre your mind.

4. Turn Towards the Right

According to TCM, the time between 5 and 7 a.m. belongs to the organs of elimination. To stimulate the process of digestion and wake up with energy, Ayurveda recommends turning to your right and getting up from bed. The yogic theory is that the right side of our body is more action-

oriented and controls active processes such as digestion. By turning right, you activate the process of elimination. Lie down towards your right for a few minutes before leaving your bed.

…cleanse and constructive processes such as digestion. By warming this, you activate the process of elimination. The [illegible] towards this right for a few minute before leaving your bed.

2

THE OUTWARD CLEANSE

Let go of the old and bring in the new. Personal hygiene is a sign of a clear mind, self-care and commitment to the day's results. It gives us physical energy to go about the day's work, along with mental stability—think about how settled you feel after a bath. For me, a cleanse extends to the purification of sense organs. Today, more than ever before, we're constantly consuming information via what we see, smell, hear and speak, both consciously and subconsciously. This constant flow of information builds up layer upon layer in our minds and filters down to the subconscious. Even without us realizing it, this data begins to change our thinking, character and intelligence. Which is why we need to purify our sense organs.

Therefore, hygiene doesn't just mean a quick wash with soap and water. It includes small practices that go beyond cleaning towards building immunity, cognitive abilities and energy.

Eyes

I would love to say I'm one of those people who just bounces out of bed. Even though I naturally wake up a little bit before 6 a.m., I feel sleepy and want to snuggle in the blanket just a little bit longer. I've tried many times to go back to sleep, but such is my body clock that I have to eventually drag myself out to face the day.

I begin my day by washing my eyes with chilled rosewater to wake myself up. Rose is an extremely cooling flower, and the eyes are the seat of pitta or fire. So rosewater (administered with eye cups or a dropper) helps calm inflammation, keeps the eyes moist and even reduces swelling and strain. I like to keep a small bottle of rosewater handy even while I write. As my work involves looking at the computer screen for most of the day, I use rosewater periodically to prevent dry eye and strain.

A lot of people also like to splash their eyes with water upon waking up. This is a wonderful practice to cleanse and refresh yourself, but I wouldn't recommend using tap water as it is contaminated. You don't want it going directly into the mucous membranes. Instead, use cool, filtered water to splash your eyes, not just in the morning but a few times a day, to reduce strain and inflammation.

If you have the time and inclination, you could also practice *nethra shuddhi*, an old ayurvedic practice to clean the eyes with either diluted rosewater or *triphala*. Because of its high-antioxidant composition of *amla*, *haritaki*, *bhibhitaki* and triphala, if consumed regularly, is beneficial for ocular diseases. Its astringent, dosha-balancing and cooling properties make it beneficial as a daily eye wash as well. A small study

found that triphala eye drops help relieve computer vision syndrome, which causes, among other things, dry, burning eyes, redness, dryness and tears.

To clean your eyes with triphala:

1. Soak a small teaspoon of triphala overnight in a cup of water.
2. Strain it in the morning using a fine mesh such as a cheesecloth or an old T-shirt.
3. Fill eye cups with this liquid till they're three-fourths full.
4. Bend your head and dip your eyes into the cup. Press the edges of the cup around the eye circumference to 'seal' them in.
5. Stay in this position, open your eyes and blink a few times. The water may feel a little uncomfortable or sting mildly. If, however, there is sharp pain or burning, stop immediately and rinse eyes with cool water.
6. If you're used to this procedure, tilt your chin up with the cup nicely sealed around the eye.
7. Open your eyes, blink a few times, then rotate your eyes in a clockwise and counter-clockwise direction to wash them properly.
8. Bend your head, remove the cups and lift your head.
9. Drain the triphala infusion and splash your eyes with cool, filtered water.

Note: It is better to use glass or ceramic cups so they don't pinch the eyes. Practice this once or twice a week, unless advised to do this daily by an ayurvedic doctor. If you're suffering from an eye disease, consult a medical professional before you try this.

In Ayurveda, hot water is never used to wash the head and eyes. These are the seat of pitta, fire, and must always be kept cool.

According to Ayurveda, a lukewarm bath is beneficial in all seasons rather than extremely chilled showers or a hot bath. This keeps your metabolism in balance.

TCM does not recommend hot water to bathe in the morning. Cooling down from a hot bath uses up yang energy, which is outwards and expansive, and which is why you feel tired afterwards. Hot baths are great in the evening but not in the morning, when you want to feel energized and fresh.

Mouth

The mouth and tongue are clear indicators of your health. It is believed in Ayurveda that each part of the tongue mirrors the health of your organs. The front sides of your tongue belong to the lungs, while the front centre is the heart. In the middle of the tongue lie the liver, spleen, pancreas and stomach, while the back of the tongue is about the lower organs such as the colon, intestines and reproductive system.

The teeth represent vata, the master dosha, which needs to be handled delicately. Therefore, teeth love gentle, soothing treatments and oil, which are all vata-pacifying. Even if you don't believe in traditional sciences, the old practices of oil pulling and tongue scraping have the ability to reduce modern-day maladies such as gingivitis, plaque and the reduction of bacterial colonies in the mouth. While brushing and flossing are undoubtedly gifts of modern living, older ayurvedic practices go beyond just oral health and affect the functioning of the entire body.

Tongue scraping

Even though you may brush your teeth before you sleep, the body detoxifies itself all night. This is why, when you wake up in the morning, there is a coating on the tongue, which is basically the toxins that the body has regurgitated overnight. The simple act of tongue scraping eliminates these toxins in a few strokes.

Many people clean the tongue with a toothbrush, assuming it would be adequate. But studies have proved that a tongue scraper provides up to 75 per cent reduction of volatile sulphur compounds (which cause bad breath) as compared to a toothbrush, which removes only 40 per cent. It was also found that this practice reduced the amount of bacteria on the tongue.

Materials and Method

In Ayurveda, different materials work for various doshas. Copper is recommended for kapha, silver is recommended for pitta and gold recommended to balance vata. Silver and gold may be impractical suggestions in the modern world. However, copper generally works for this practice as it is naturally an anti-bacterial metal. Stainless steel is another great option, which suits all dosha types. Both copper and steel tongue scrapers are easily available.

To do:

✿ This must be practised after brushing teeth and before oil pulling.

✿ Wash your tongue cleaner and use it to scrape the centre, sides and the back of your tongue.

✿ Use light, even strokes, about ten to twelve in number.

✿ Make sure you scrape the back of the tongue, since that is connected to the colon. You will get a mild retching sensation, but according to Ayurveda, this stimulates peristalsis, which leads to better elimination.

✿ Clean thoroughly and store.

Oil Pulling

Despite popular opinion, there is no conclusive evidence to prove that the practice of oil pulling helps reduce migraine, acne or enhance immunity. However, when practised over a period of time, you will find an improvement in oral hygiene. I can speak only from personal experience, but I have found that this is a deeply detoxifying practice that enhances gum and tooth health. I have one tooth that hurts mildly when I stop oil pulling. When I begin again, the pain somewhat disappears. I'm not saying this could be a replacement for a filling or a root canal surgery, but I do feel that this could perhaps delay these procedures.

There are oils are that are mainly spoken about when it comes to this practice. Traditionally, sesame oil was used for oil pulling for its warming, anti-bacterial and vata-pacifying qualities. I have mentioned previously that the teeth are a location for vata. Therefore, according to Ayurveda, since sesame oil is the best to balance this dosha, it makes teeth strong and healthy. In fact, it is also recommended that after brushing, one must chew a small handful of roasted sesame seeds to improve oral health.

Coconut oil is a modern-day recommendation for oil pulling. A lot of it has to do with its sudden status as a superfood. Lobbyists have positioned this oil as the ultimate solution for health, whether you add a teaspoon to your coffee or use it for oil pulling. In Ayurveda, coconut oil is cooling and pacifying, it reduces inflammation, including that of the gums, and nourishes the tissues. Traditionally, though, it wasn't suggested for oil pulling.

I have used both oils and enjoy them for different reasons. Coconut oil is great for summer, when it is naturally in a liquid state. We cannot ignore that this oil also has anti-fungal attributes, which are beneficial for oral health. Additionally, I find that coconut oil also helps whiten the teeth a tiny bit as compared to sesame. Perhaps this has something to do with the presence of lauric acid.

Sesame oil is a little bit thicker, therefore it is better to 'pull' impurities as compared to coconut, which is runnier. Its warming nature makes it more suitable during the winter months, when it is more convenient to use since it doesn't freeze. I also prefer massaging this over my gums because of its dense, emollient texture.

Personally, I like to use coconut oil in the morning, when I practise this for longer (about 20 minutes). Sesame oil is used in the evening, when I use it for a quick swish (less than a minute) before I spit it out. You absolutely do not have to do this twice a day. I mention this as an optional practice for those who may have such an inclination.

Ghee Pulling

For those with chronic hyperacidity or acid reflux, Ayurveda recommends ghee pulling, wherein small pieces of *mishri* are chewed with a teaspoon of ghee, mixed together with the saliva, swished through the mouth and then ingested. This reduces pitta and is good for healing mouth and gastric ulcers.

Astringent Mouth Rinse

If you want to avoid oil completely, you can also do a mouth rinse with triphala tea. If you are preparing triphala to clean your eyes, you can use the leftover liquid as a mouthwash. The astringent and antimicrobial qualities of triphala extract impurities, which makes it an effective daily mouth rinse. In fact, there is some data to show that a triphala rinse may be comparable to chlorhexidine to reduce tooth mobility, bleeding gums and sensitivity. To prepare triphala tea, soak 1 teaspoon powder overnight in a cup of water or add a teaspoon to a cup of hot water in the morning. Let it cool before use.

Oil Pulling 101

- ✿ Sip about a tablespoon of oil and swish it around the mouth, making sure it goes through all the spaces between the teeth.
- ✿ You can begin to practise this for 5 minutes. The oil will turn thick and creamy. Spit it out into a bin and not the basin to prevent clogging.
- ✿ Rinse with warm water.
- ✿ The correct sequence is: first, brush your teeth, then scrape your tongue and finally, perform oil pulling. First, the surface must be cleaned, and then oil pulling will remove deeper toxins from the oral cavity.
- ✿ Take care not to swallow the oil since it is full of plaque and microbes that have been extracted.

✿ Do not eat or drink anything till the oral cavity is clean with these practices.

Nose

The nostrils are the gateway to the brain. Scientists are studying intranasal administration of medicines to see how drugs can travel from the nasal mucosa to the brain and bloodstream. Within the scope of yoga and Ayurveda, the nostrils are of great significance since they hold *ida* and pingala, the two main etheric channels or nadis. The word nadi comes from *nad*, which means vibration. The right nostril, called the pingala, stands for our active side, whereas the ida or the left nostril, for our more passive characteristics. A balance between these etheric channels means a balanced mind and body.

Two main practices are recommended to clear these channels. The practice of *jal neti* involves pouring warm saline water down each nostril and out from the other. Nasya, on the other hand, mainly involves pouring a few drops of oil down the nostrils. Both practices have benefits and boost immunity, keep the nasal channels clear and calm the mind. Ayurveda says that nasya, particularly, helps the brain because fatty substances such as oil help cross the blood-brain barrier and deliver medicine directly.

Neti

I first learnt jal neti at an ayurvedic spa. Because I was suffering from migraines, their in-house vaidya recommended jal neti. I have found it to be fairly effective in the treatment of

migraines, but only when done just when the pain begins. Additionally, I find the regular practice of neti followed by pranayama greatly reduces the incidence of infections such as the common cold. Having said that, I do not want to give instructions for jal neti as it must be learnt in person with a yoga teacher. If you're already practising nasal irrigation, these are the pointers to keep in mind:

✿ The water must be lukewarm, like your body temperature, and should be salty like your tears. Too much salt, or undissolved salt crystals, will give you a burning sensation in your nose.

✿ Only use filtered water and a good quality salt (none of the commercial iodized brands) because this will be poured into the nasal cavity.

✿ The stream of water should not flow down the face and cheeks. Instead, it must come out straight, like a thread.

✿ Make sure you finish by closing one nostril and forcefully exhaling (like in *kapalabhanti*) with your head tilted towards one side. Do both sides and then bend forward and exhale sharply with both nostrils. This is to ensure that all the water is drained out.

✿ Check if any water is left behind by forcefully exhaling on the back of your palm. If there are droplets, do more rounds of the forceful exhalations till the breath comes out clear.

Nasya

My first experience of this practice was during a twenty-one-day panchakarma or the full ayurvedic detox. There are many

different types of nasya therapies. During my panchakarma, my nasya was followed up with *dhumpan*, where I inhaled smoke from a medicated cloth. But at home, nasya is much simpler and easier than jal neti. It's just the mental block that prevents you from pouring oil into nostrils.

.The safest at-home daily practice is called *pratimarsha* nasya, where the little finger is dipped in oil and inserted within the nostril. Beneficial for the health of the neck, head and oral cavity, this type of nasya can be practised every day, at any age and during all seasons. In Ayurveda, this practice is believed to prevent respiratory allergies, stop hair from greying, enhance immunity, relieve fatigue and is also good for cervical spondylosis or stiffness of the neck.

Even though the benefits of pratimarsha nasya go beyond protection of the mucous membranes, scientific papers describe clearly how oils can form a barrier against environmental pollution. Because most pollutants are lipid or fat insoluble, coating the mucous membranes of the nose forms the first line of defence against pollution. Nasya also increases the bioavailability of medicine in the plasma. Small studies have shown the daily practice of nasya to be beneficial for various conditions, including migraines, allergies and even insomnia.

While pratimarsha nasya can be practised with just sesame oil or ghee, the ayurvedic preparation of *anu thailam* is recommended by most vaidyas. Made with a multitude of ingredients, including wood apple, lotus, sandalwood, *shatavari*, cinnamon, cardamom, sesame oil and goat milk, this oil is supposed to improve conditions of the head, neck and shoulders. Be careful when administering this oil, as it is very potent. Start by just applying it on the insides of the

nostril with a finger and when you're comfortable, use no more than a drop or two on a regular basis.

To do:

- ✿ Lie down on the bed, without a pillow. You can even lie on the edge so that the head dips lower than the nostrils.
- ✿ Tilt your chin up and release one or two drops of oil in each nostril.
- ✿ Pinch the nostrils and inhale sharply.
- ✿ You can also practise this sitting up. Dip your little finger into the oil. Insert it into one nostril and sniff the oil. Repeat on the other.
- ✿ You might get a postnasal drip in the throat—make sure you spit it out.
- ✿ Personally, I don't like to practise jal neti and nasya on the same day. I practise each, every alternate day.

Note: If you have respiratory conditions or any other chronic disease, consult your physician before practising this. Avoid after drinking alcohol.

Ears

A healer once told me that our sense of hearing takes us closest to the divine, and our sense of sight takes us furthest away. I don't know whether this is true or not, but I do know that music has the ability to heal us and listening has the ability to teach us new things. Ayurveda says that loss of hearing is caused due to an imbalance in the vata dosha, which is the

humour of air and space. It is believed that the skin and bones of the ear become dry, thereby affecting the hearing. Because vata has dry qualities that are pacified with oils, therefore, an ear massage/oiling is highly recommended. However, before you attempt this ritual, you must check with an ENT surgeon to confirm that you do not have perforation of the eardrum. If you do, please avoid this ritual.

The ayurvedic therapy for ear problems is *karna purana*, which literally means filling the ear with oil. However, this too must be practised with guidance from an ayurvedic doctor. To protect your ears on a daily basis, apply a little bit of oil on your little finger and rub gently around the ear canal. Do not apply too much pressure. If you have time, rub some oil onto the rest of the ear.

To do:

☼ Ideally, this must be done after massaging the entire head. Therefore, it can be seen as a weekly ritual, part of your weekend *champi*.

☼ After massaging your head, pour three to four drops of oil into one ear. Then close the flap and gently massage the centre of the ear.

☼ The acupressure points within the ear lie behind the ear lobe (wind screen); the deepest part of the cartilage within the ear (daith); the top of the ear (ear apex); and the point in the centre of the ear where it connects to the face (ear gate). Use firm pressure to massage these points.

☼ Lie on your side for 15 minutes and then repeat on the other side.

Skin and Hair

In earlier times, when we lived at a more leisurely pace, baths weren't just about cleaning the body but also an opportunity to socialize with friends. In the *jimjilbangs* of South Korea and *onsens* in Japan, this culture still persists. Japanese and Korean women thoroughly scrub and soap themselves *before* they step into the hot, mineral-rich waters that are therapeutic and not just cleansing. Of course, on a daily basis, we don't have the time for such luxuries. In the morning it's all about convenience—a quick shower at the most.

Most people talk about energizing or 'waking up' the skin with a shower. However, the skin is a nocturnal creature that performs its duties of cell renewal at night. It's because of this reason that, for most people, their skin looks best in the morning. Still, as you're exposed to environmental pollutants and internal stress during the day, the morning prep must support, protect and set you up for several hours.

Face Cleanse

After your skin has worked hard the entire night to work at a cellular level, it seems unfair to wash it with a harsh, foaming cleanser. Women with the most beautiful skin have often told me that they never use soap on their face. Admittedly, there are times, especially during the humid months, when nothing feels as good as a foaming cleanser. Still, cleansing should not strip the skin of its natural oils, no matter what your age may be. In fact, with a dry herb/clay cleanser, you can even squeeze in a quick 2-minute

mask before you get to work. Natural cleansers include oils for dry, raw honey for normal and clay for oily skin. Leave each ingredient on for between 2-5 minutes before you wash it off.

Clay

While oil and honey can be left on the skin indefinitely, clay must only be used for no more than a few minutes. Clay works especially well during monsoon. If you're prone to a heat rash it calms and dries it down. I like to mix my clay (usually kaolin or bentonite for me) with chilled rosewater. *Multani mitti* works better for oily complexions and kaolin clay for skin that's dry and sensitive. If you want to leave clay on your face for longer periods, mix it with honey and water. The honey will prevent the clay from becoming completely dry and therefore irritating your skin.

Honey

There's nothing more healing for the skin than raw honey. Honey is antibacterial, antifungal and anti-inflammatory. It contains enzymes, organic acids, peptides and antioxidants such as such as phenolic acids and flavonoids, all of which benefit the skin. The best part is that it works as a humectant, meaning that it draws moisture into the skin. Its dense, sticky texture ensures that it deep-cleans your skin, but without dehydration. It doesn't spread easily on the skin, but to increase spread-ability, apply it on a damp face, or spritz rosewater before application. I like to keep the honey on

my face while I'm brushing my teeth or oil pulling so that I maximize it during this time, keeping it on my face as a mask. Wash it off while you shower.

Oil

To soothe dry, parched skin, oil works well as a cleanser. Jojoba is the lightest oil since it resembles the skin's sebum. Almond oil is richer as it contains high amounts of vitamin E. Even apricot oil is good for cleansing—it contains less vitamin E than almond but about 70 per cent oleic acid, which is known for its hydrating and anti-inflammatory properties. The other oils suited to cleansing are sunflower, olive and grapeseed for their lightweight texture.

To utilize oil as cleanser, apply it all over the face, neck and décolletage, massaging in upward strokes. Then remove with a hot towel or a muslin washcloth to really clean out the pores. I find that oil cleansing is better suited for the evening, when you want to remove layers of sunscreen, skincare and makeup. In the morning, clay or honey work better when you're in a rush.

Yoghurt

Rich in probiotics, lactic acids and emollients, yoghurt can be used as both a cleanser and a face mask. Especially on heated, sun-exposed skin, the application of chilled, full-fat and preferably homemade yoghurt can calm and soothe the skin. I learned to use yogurt from Anuska, my yoga teacher,

who used the water on top of homemade yoghurt as a face toner, and the thicker, milky part as a face mask. She said that when skincare was unavailable in war-torn Bosnia, this would be their one and only skincare.

All-Natural Double Cleansing for Mature Skin

This works beautifully towards the end of the day; however, it is suitable for those who only wear skincare, as it may not be able to remove heavy make-up.

Step 1: Dip a cotton wool in cold/warm whole milk and wipe the entire face and neck. You could also pour some milk into the palm of your hand and massage it all over the face and neck. Then wipe off with a damp, hot towel.

Step 2: Massage some raw honey into your face and neck. Pat a little bit of water into it to 'emulsify' and spread the honey. Then when it's massaged in well, remove it with a damp, hot washcloth.

(Note: If you have oily skin, you may want to replace the milk with yoghurt.)

Daily Cleansing Paste for All Skin Types

¼ tsp *kasturi manjal* (wild turmeric)
1/4 tsp red sandalwood
1/4 tsp orange peel
1/4 tsp raw honey/yoghurt
1 tsp oatmeal (avoid this if your skin is very dry)
Rosewater/honey/milk to make a paste (you can mix all three)

Method:

✿ Mix all the ingredients and apply over the face and neck.

✿ If you have time in the morning, then allow it to semi-dry.

✿ Wet skin with a bit of water and gently rub off in circular strokes.

✿ If you are only using this paste for cleansing, then skip the red sandalwood, since it is a precious ingredient. Add it when you have 10 minutes to apply on your face.

✿ Unless you have very sensitive skin, this can be used every day. It gently exfoliates, brightens the skin and leaves it clean without over-drying.

✿ If you use very strong retinols and peels, avoid this. Instead, only use raw honey to clean your face.

Healing Cleansing Paste for Acneic skin

1 tsp *lodhra* powder
1 tsp *mulethi* (licorice) powder
½ tsp *gotu kola* (centella asiatica) powder
½ tsp raw honey
Rosewater to make into a paste

Method:

✿ Lodhra powder is recommended by Ayurveda for its anti-acne properties. It cools overheated skin and its calming nature is enhanced when it is soaked in a silver bowl. If you remember and have the time, mix this with rosewater in a silver container and refrigerate overnight.

✿ Mulethi is revered for its scar-healing abilities and gotu kola for its wound-healing properties.

✿ Use it in the morning as a cleanser by adding a bit of honey to heal and hydrate the skin. Skip honey if you're vegan.

Detoxifying Cleansing Paste for Oily Skin

½ tsp neem powder
½ tsp amla powder
1 tsp mung dal flour
Rosewater to make into paste

Method:

✿ Neem is antibacterial and therefore beneficial for oily, acne-prone skin; amla gives a shot of vitamin C for glow; mung flour works as a mild astringent.

✿ Mix together with a bit of rosewater and apply till the paste is semi-dry. Wash off. Do not rub on active breakouts.

✿ This paste is only for oily skin.

Smoothing Cleansing Paste for Mature Skin

2 tbsp masoor dal (red lentil) paste
2 tbsp white sesame seed paste
Raw milk (infused with a pinch of saffron) to bind

Method:

✿ Masoor dal works better than *besan* to exfoliate skin as it is more mucilaginous, which makes it

less drying. The fat from sesame seeds works as an emollient on the skin. Soak both overnight in milk.

☼ Infuse a few threads of saffron in it till it turns a yellow colour and then soak masoor dal and white sesame seeds.

☼ Grind to a paste in the morning. Add extra milk if the paste is too dense.

☼ Pat all over the face. Rub off when semi-dry.

☼ You can make a small batch for four to five days and refrigerate.

☼ Do not rub if you are using strong retinols and peels.

Body Cleanse

There is no doubt that a bath invigorates the body, awakens the senses and alerts the mind. But some get lazy, especially during the weekend, about the daily ritual of bathing. But if you understand how a bath works, you'll know it goes beyond just aesthetics, positively impacting health and wellness every single day.

According to the ayurvedic system, it is believed that if you eat healthy, have a clean lifestyle and follow circadian rhythms, your body will work very hard during the night to detoxify every organ. This detoxification happens in many different ways. Your stool, sweat and urine are the primary waste materials or *malas*. However, the secretions from the eyes and other mucous membranes, the coating on your tongue and the oil on the skin are also waste thrown out from your body.

Because each and every cell in your body detoxifies during the night, your morning shower isn't just about grooming and getting ready for the day. In its deeper relevance, your morning bath removes all the secretions that have been released through the night.

The Morning Bath

Everything is interconnected in traditional sciences, therefore, baths too cannot be viewed in isolation. Here are a few pointers to be kept in mind:

1. Never bathe right after a meal because it dampens the digestive fire, which means your food will not be metabolized optimally. Either do it before you eat, or 25-30 minutes after a meal.
2. Lukewarm water is considered to be the best for bathing. In summer, this lukewarm will be slightly cooler, while in winter it will be slightly warmer. Hot baths are only for the sick, the old or the very young. Even though TCM recommends cold showers, Ayurveda suggests they're best avoided since the coldness imbalances the metabolic fire. The jury is still out on this one, since cold showers and cryotherapy have proved to be beneficial in many conditions, including for muscle healing and weight loss. Ultimately, we all have to decide what works for us.
3. Even though Ayurveda may not recommend cold showers in general, it is recommended that the head and eyes must always be washed with cool water. The eyes are the seat of pitta or fire, therefore cool water is said to invigorate and revive their functioning.

4. Additionally, bathing in cold water during winter enrages kapha and vata, while utilizing hot water during the summer will agitate the blood and pitta.

5. A body massage in the morning before a bath is supposed to be grounding for the mind. While I have tried a pre-bath massage, I find it impractical in the modern world, though ultimately it's just a question of building habit. For me, the morning bath has to be quick, cleansing and fuss-free. Therefore, I like to rub in a cold-pressed oil after my bath on damp skin.

Body Cleansing Powder

1 tbsp khus powder (Indian Vetiver)
1 tbsp *anantmool* powder (sarsaparilla)
1 cup *navara* red rice powder/red rice powder
½ cup masoor dal powder
1 tbsp saunf (fennel seed) powder
1 tbsp green cardamom powder or sandalwood powder
½ tsp almond oil (optional)
½ tsp honey (optional)
Hot milk/green tea/yoghurt/aloe vera gel to bind

Method:

Mix all the powders in the medium of your choice. I prefer hot milk since I have dry skin. Make a thin paste and use this to clean the body. You can also leave it on as a body mask (but make sure the paste is thicker) when you have the time.

Hair Cleanse

Modern aesthetics leave little room for traditional remedies. Hair is a classic example. The current aesthetic of hair is shiny, freshly shampooed and blow-dried. We are repulsed by the smell and texture of hair oil, even though it may benefit hair growth. Traditional hair rituals such as oiling and henna are being replaced with synthetic colours and hair spas. But I have seen the benefits of ancestral wisdom first hand. While current aesthetics are relevant to the modern world, it is foolish not to utilize the knowledge we have culturally.

For many years, I'd shampoo my hair almost every day. I wanted it to look a certain way, which could only be afforded when I would wash it regularly. During those years, I would always get a flaky scalp during the changing seasons. This flakiness also affected my skin, which became irritated for a couple of months every year. But then I began oiling my hair before every shampoo and washed it only a few times in the week.

These days, I wash my hair twice a week. After doing this regularly for years, my scalp stopped reacting to the change of seasons. There's no more flakiness, my hair has stopped falling and is in the best health. My experience is that hair loves simplicity. An excess of synthetic colour, excessive shampooing, multiple products and heat styling will break down its structure and irritate the scalp.

Studies have shown that herbal hair oils made with ingredients such as amla, *brahmi*, fenugreek seeds and hibiscus provide results in terms of hair thickness and growth, comparable to minoxidil. Even if you don't want to keep

the oil overnight, 20-30 minutes is enough. Just don't use cooling oils such as coconut during winter because they make you susceptible to colds.

Softening Hair Cleansing Powder

1 cup *arappu* tree powder
½ cup *shikakai* powder
½ cup amla powder
¼ cup *reetha* powder (if hair is oiled)
or
1/4 cup mung powder if hair isn't oiled
1 heaped tsp hibiscus powder

Method:

This is an adaptation of a traditional recipe. Mix all together and store. To use, mix a couple of heaped teaspoons (or more depending on hair length). Let it soak for a while. Then add more water to make a runny paste and rub it all over your scalp.

Cleansing Powder for Oily Hair

Mix equal parts hibiscus, neem, amla and mung dal powders in some water. Let it soak for 10-15 minutes and then make a runny paste to cleanse your hair.

3

DAYTIME ELIXIRS

The real beauty of the early morning elixir isn't the fact that it fills us to the brim with health. For most of us it brings with it hope and an expectation that this drink will help resolve long-standing conditions, purify the body and transform skin. We may not be entirely wrong either. Your morning drink could help reduce bloat, kick-start metabolism, detoxify, alkalize or hydrate the body. The highly individualized, ritualistic tendencies of the morning beverage make it the most sustainable health habit.

I like to rotate my morning elixirs depending on the season. If I have an ayurvedic prescription, it takes precedence, followed by other juices and teas. The thing with morning elixirs is that you needn't choose just one. If you follow the ayurveda food rules, you know that the main meal is around 12 p.m. This is because the digestive fire burns bright around this time. My ayurvedic doctor likes to compare the stomach to a *havan kund*. If the fire isn't burning bright, whatever offering you will put in will not burn properly. Similarly, if

you consume food at a time when the digestive fire is not at its peak, it will not digest properly.

I eat my first big meal around lunch so I can consume a few health boosters before. The first is an ayurvedic *churna* with detoxifying herbs followed by green powders dissolved in water, and then some sort of fat. In winter, the fat would be green tea with coconut oil and in summer I like to drink raw mango *panna* in which I add two tablespoons of pre-soaked chia seeds. In addition to this, I enjoy a couple of portions of fresh fruit and a cup or two of herbal tea. Maybe some muesli if I'm writing, because carbs fuel my mind. If you have the time and inclination, try to keep a gap of half an hour between every drink and fruits. I like every ingredient to work independently before another can be added. This is what is recommended in Ayurveda and it works well for me.

Detoxifying Elixirs

Mornings are special because the mind is clear and body feels fresh, therefore more receptive. Detoxification is a natural process for the body, but certain spices and herbs can accelerate that process. The simplest way to detoxify is a glass of hot water. Of course, there is the age-old recipe of lemon and honey, but it may not suit everyone, especially pitta types prone to hyperacidity.

When I speak of detoxifiers, I mean foods and herbs that have the ability to purify the body internally. They could work by purifying the blood, clearing the liver or helping it work better—one way or another, they need to have a deeply

cleansing effect so that anything consumed afterwards will get beautifully absorbed into the body.

✿ Nettle

I first came across nettle a couple of decades ago. I discovered that it was utilized as a leafy vegetable and a drink by Chinese herbalists and zen masters rumoured to live well over a 100 years. In Europe, it is used to treat urinary problems. When I consumed it regularly as tea in my twenties, I found that it helped keep my skin clear and also helped reduce rosacea.

Nettle is a weed, and like any ingredient that grows freely, it's also packed with nutrients. In fact, any ingredient which grows on its own is more nutrient-dense than farmed produce. Despite its uses in traditional and folk medicine, nettle isn't well-researched. But that doesn't mean it isn't worth a second glance. In a small study on fish, it was found that when nettle was given as a part of the diet, their immunity improved and they became more resistant towards microbes. Another animal study found that it did indeed have liver-protective properties. Nettle leaf also encourages the renewal of intestinal villi or tiny finger-like projections that run along the entire intestines. The villi absorb nutrition from food and pass it on to the bloodstream. Additionally, nettle helps in eliminating harmful bacteria from the urinary tract, reduces inflammation and helps control high blood glucose levels.

Take a small teaspoon of dried leaves (or one teabag). Pour over freshly boiled water. Let brew for at least 10 minutes to extract all the properties of nettle. Sip either first thing in the

morning 15 minutes after drinking a glass of warm water, or between meals.

Indian Sarsaparilla

Chronic skin problems such as acne, eczema and psoriasis are clearly reflective of poor-quality blood. This herb, also known as anantmool, *nannari* or *sariva*, is one of the best blood purifiers in Ayurveda and is considered to be the best remedy for chronic skin conditions. In fact, my morning ayurvedic powder also contains this herb, which keeps my skin clear despite being on synthetic hormones. Anantmool is loved because it cools the body, brings down inflammation and also works as a diuretic, thereby reducing water retention.

Because it eliminates excess heat from the body, it calms an angry, disturbed mind. Studies have also shown that it has potent antimicrobial activities against bacteria such as E. Coli and salmonella. It helps reduce liver toxicity and increases positive markers such as liver collagen and ascorbic acid. It is also anti-arthritic, antipsychotic, anti-acne and wound healing. It's no surprise then that it is considered to be the panacea for skin relief. Lastly, the saponins in this herb increase the bioavailability or absorption of other supplements in the body.

Anantmool must ideally be consumed with just water. You can either consume a small teaspoon with warm water or brew it as a 'tea' by brewing the powder in hot water for 10 minutes. The tea is quite fragrant—to elevate the taste further, add a teaspoon of raw honey when it cools a bit. You can drink this first thing in the morning or between meals.

☼ Neem

Bitter is considered to be the most detoxifying taste in Ayurveda. It is the flavour that helps clear the liver, especially if consumed during spring. Bitter is also the most cooling taste out of all the six flavours in Ayurveda. In TCM, bitter herbs have a cleansing action, which directly impacts the heart. It is also supposed to dry dampness, therefore it helps reduce mucous production, which is associated with inflammation and infection.

Traditionally, in India, we consume five *neem kay kopal* or the slightly reddish baby neem leaves for a period of three weeks on an empty stomach. In a healthy human, this is supposed to detoxify the body for a full year. You can also consume neem leaves by crushing one or two in a cup of hot water and drinking it as a 'tea' after meals. Care must be taken, however, not to consume neem for more than a couple of months. Since neem has insecticidal properties, consumed over a long period, it kills even the healthy bacteria in the gut.

☼ Amla

The Indian gooseberry is well-loved for its antioxidant properties. Being one of the richest sources of vitamin C, it is utilized for its anti-ageing properties by both traditional and western medicine. The best part about amla is that unlike vitamin C from citrus fruits (that degrades very easily), the vitamin C from Indian gooseberry isn't sensitive to light or heat. This means you can pickle, cook, juice and powder this berry without fear of ruining its nutritional profile.

Even though its biggest strength is its rejuvenating power, amla works wonderfully as a detoxifier as well. In Ayurveda and Tibetan medicine, it is known for its cooling properties. It also strengthens digestion, helps with the absorption of calcium, deeply detoxifies the tissues, promotes healthy hair and strong teeth, cures anaemia, boosts immunity and slows ageing. When in doubt, choose amla for its rejuvenating, fortifying and detoxifying qualities.

The Indian gooseberry can be consumed in many different ways. There is no doubt that freshly squeezed juice is the best option. However, I prefer not to get rid of the fibrous pulp. Therefore, grate fresh, mix both the pulp and juice in a quarter glass of water and drink up. You could also consume grated amla with a teaspoon of raw honey in winter. If you have amla powder, you can add it to smoothies and green juices. Amla powder/dried berries can also be brewed into herbal tea that can be enjoyed at any time of the day.

✿ Beetroot

The juice of this root vegetable is common during winter, when it's in season, usually combined with carrot and ginger, makes it a nutrition bomb with a powerhouse of nutrients like folates, vitamin C, iron, vitamin A and B vitamins. But did you know that beetroots are highly therapeutic on their own? I learnt about the healing power of beets at a health spa where residents were given fresh beet juice first thing in the morning for its ability to clear the intestines. This is because these vegetables are rich in betaine, which is known to balance stomach acids and improve digestion.

In TCM, they're supposed to help strengthen the heart and calm the spirit. They're also utilized for their ability to detoxify the liver, purify the blood and lubricate the intestines. Studies have shown that beets help lower blood pressure, reduce blood glucose and help in cases of kidney dysfunction. They're also rich in compounds called nitrates, that convert into nitric oxide and help increase blood flow to the brain. When combined with exercise, these nitrates also help improve stamina and endurance.

Beetroot juice is safe for most people; however, if you are prone to kidney stones, then check with your doctor before consuming them. Also, only eat/juice them during winter when they're in season. According to Ayurveda, they're warming in nature, therefore unsuitable for the hot weather or for very high pitta types. One cup of juice is safe for daily consumption.

Alkalizing Elixirs

The body is a beautifully designed machine, quite capable of being in a perfect balance of alkalinity and acidity. A pH of 0 is considered highly acidic, while a pH of 14 highly alkaline. The normal pH of the blood lies between 7.35 and 7.45. Modern lifestyles and poor eating habits such as too much meat, processed food, preservatives, refined carbohydrates and sugar have disturbed this natural balance of the body. Over time, with continued abuse, the body becomes acidic with increased inflammation, which leads to chronic disease.

When acids accumulate in the body, it cannot naturally neutralize them if there is an overload of toxins. To dissolve

these acids, it leaches minerals from bones and joints, which eventually leads to osteoporosis. To counter this, it also tries to protect itself by increasing fat storage. An acidic body is the perfect host for bad bacteria, yeast and viruses that thrive in such an environment. Signs of internal inflammation include but are not limited to fatigue, digestive issues, aches, pains, migraines, bad breath and fungal infections.

Even though the problem looks complicated, the solution could be as simple as adding more plant-based foods. Fruits and vegetables are in fact the number one alkalizers of the body. Cooling fruits such as apples, melons, bananas, grapes and pears, along with green leafy vegetables, sweet potatoes, cruciferous vegetables, cold pressed oils, nuts and seeds, all help alkalize the body. Add to this stress-reducing activities, such as deep breathing, which also help bring down the acidic load. An early morning addition of greens is part of the alkalization process.

✿ Wheat and Barley Grass

In TCM, cereal grasses such as wheat and barley are revered for their cooling and cleansing properties. While fresh juice from the shoots of the seeds is always preferred, I also find it convenient to use powders. The nutritional profile of wheat and barley grass is sort of the same. The antioxidant profile of barley grass is higher, while the total phenolic composition and flavonoids are much higher in wheatgrass. Antioxidants are molecules that help fight cell-damaging free radicals. Phenolic compounds and flavonoids have antioxidant properties but are used by the body for specific actions. For

instance, anthocyanins in blueberries give them their colour and work as powerful antioxidants.

In both these grasses, the chlorophyll binds with carcinogens and hinders their access to our cells. In addition, they also contain superoxide dismutase, a powerful antioxidant, along with saponarin and gamma-aminobutyric acid (GABA), which help bring down inflammation.

Barley grass helps prevent chronic diseases, reduces inflammation, alkalizes the body and helps with weight loss, while the tryptophan content also helps enhance sleep. Wheatgrass has slightly a lower amount of nutrients but is greatly valued for its benefits towards blood-related diseases such as thalassemia. Personally, the big difference for me is that wheatgrass is slightly mild in flavour, whereas barley grass is sharper and more bitter.

I also like to rotate both by consuming each for a period of two months. I add 1 tablespoon of cereal grass powder into half a cup of water, so as not to dilute the nutrients with too much water. You can drink this first thing in the morning on an empty stomach or between meals. If you have fresh wheat and barley grass but find them painful to juice, eat the whole grass, which will also give you the additional fibre.

✿ Moringa

I love moringa not only for its high nutritional profile but also because it is one of the most sustainable trees. It grows freely, without much food and water. It's not surprising that it is used to help children suffering from malnutrition in cash-strapped economies around the world. Just like amla,

moringa's nutrients are not prone to degradation with heat and light. Therefore, the powder can be kept stored and the fresh leaves cooked without fear of losing its precious vitamins and minerals.

Moringa is a favourite green powder among nutritionists because it can be used for supplementation. It is a powerhouse of nutrients—just 6 spoonsful will enable a woman to get the required daily amount of calcium and iron during pregnancy. To prevent an overdose of iron, consume moringa powder in low doses. Even though research papers recommend a maximum of 70 gm a day, I like to consume no more than 1 heaped tablespoon in a small amount of water every day. Again, I prefer to rotate between the cereal grasses and moringa, so that I don't consume any one of these potent nutraceuticals continuously over the long term.

✿ Spirulina

This ancient microalga was also eaten as food by the Mayans, with its unusually high protein content (60–70 per cent by dry weight) and rich profile of vitamins, minerals, enzymes and phytonutrients. The cholesterol-lowering abilities of this super green are documented via animal studies, along with its ability to prevent fatty liver. Spirulina also has potent antioxidant and anti-inflammatory properties; however, care must be taken that all green powders must be consumed after a thorough evaluation with your doctor and from clean, organic sources.

Microalgae such as spirulina are loved for their high protein content. In Chinese medicine, it is especially

beneficial for those who suffer the consequences of being on a diet full of animal fat. The gamma linoleic acid (GLA) in it helps balance hormones and calm inflammation. A daily dose of 1 teaspoon is safe to consume on a daily basis. However, those with thyroid, an autoimmune condition, kidney stones, gout, phenylketonuria or pregnant women must only consume it after consulting with a health professional.

Digestive Elixirs

The first step to healthy living is daily evacuation. This everyday habit has a lot to do with mental health, diet and how attentive we are during meals. Rushing though dinner, paying more attention to the phone than your meals will ensure that food doesn't get digested properly. We cannot carry toxins and waste material generated at night during the day. If we don't have a daily bowel movement, some of those toxins get reabsorbed into the body.

It is a well-known fact that even hormones such as oestrogen are thrown out of the body via daily elimination. Every healthy routine must begin after we clear the waste. These ingredients may help keep you regular.

✿ Chia

For morning drinks, I like to use seeds that have a bit of mucilage. This mucilage, which is basically the slippery texture and fats in the seeds, help coat and repair the lining of the stomach, which can be destroyed by antibiotics, autoimmune disorders and poor eating habits. The fat and

mucilage in these seeds also helps with better elimination, as they work as mild laxatives and help bulk up stool with the fibre content.

For a food that has a better antioxidant profile than blueberries, chia seeds are strangely marketed only for their ability to reduce weight. While the research on chia's connection with weight is inconclusive, one study proved that just 30 gm of chia seeds, taken daily with bread, reduced the sugar spike seen after meals. The seeds have also proven to be an ally for those with heart disease as they lower blood pressure and reduce the risk of heart problems. Chia contains a large amount of fibre, which can absorb up to 15 times its weight in water. This helps slow down the digestion process and the release of glucose, increases the peristaltic movement of the intestines and reduces cholesterol.

The recommended dose of chia is about 15 gm, about 1 tablespoon a day. Soak it overnight in cup of water and then drink in the morning. Chia doesn't suit everyone—if you feel that it overstimulates your digestion, it may not be right for you.

✿ Flax

Unlike many nuts and seeds that are new additions to the superfood arsenal, flax has been around for long with solid benefits that are backed by research. It is one of the best sources of ALA (alpha linolenic acid) plant-based Omega 3 fatty acids—the plant variation of Omega 3 is called alpha linoleic acid. While ALA is undoubtedly beneficial for a variety of health problems, the downside is that it makes

flax go rancid very fast. This means that it must be bought in small batches and consumed quickly. The same goes for walnuts, which also spoil rapidly because of their high fatty acid content.

Studies have shown that flaxseed has the ability to reduce blood pressure and blood glucose, and has also been utilized for a variety of cancers as a complementary supplement along with mainstream treatment. Mostly, it has been studied in its protective role against breast cancer—small human trials have shown that it protects and reduces mortality in women with breast cancer. In these studies, the recommended daily dose was 25 gm a day of milled flaxseed, or a little less than 2 tablespoons. Like all foods rich in fatty acids, these too have shown a positive effect on brain function. Additionally, the phytoestrogens in them provide oestrogenic action, which helps reduce menopausal symptoms. The dosage for postmenopausal women in the study was 40 gm (2 1/2 tablespoons) a day for a year.

The best way to consume it is when it's bought whole, then roasted and ground at home. Since this seed is prone to rancidity, avoid pre-milled powders and instead choose to mill them in the spice grinder. You can consume it with warm water but it can also be added to rotis, cakes or sprinkled over salads. Just make sure you chew the seeds thoroughly if you're eating them whole.

✡ Sabja

Basil or *sabja* seeds are often confused with chia, but, energetically, they're a little different. Chia is warming while

sabja is cooling, making them the preferred option for summer. While sabja seeds too have fatty acids, they're appreciated more for their high mineral and antioxidant content, with high levels of iron, zinc, magnesium and calcium.

Because they have the ability to expand with water, sabja seeds give you the feeling of fullness for longer. Additionally, it is said that just a teaspoon of sabja seeds contains more fibre than a whole bulb of lettuce. Because of their cooling effect on the body, these seeds are suitable for anyone with burning sensations such as hyperacidity. You can consume them with sherbet to enhance their cooling effect or soak in water and chew thoroughly. Consume no more than two teaspoons a day, after they have been soaked for 30 minutes – 3 hours.

Water Infusions

The simplest way to purify, energize and focus is to keep ourselves well hydrated. Even minor amounts of dehydration can cause a feeling of lethargy and irritability. But the ayurvedic belief is that over-drinking water can tax the kidneys. The ideal amount of water in a day comes to about 2 litres. Of course, if you stay in a hot and humid environment or work out a lot, you'll require more. It is better to drink warm or room temperature instead of cold water, because warmer water helps improve digestion and detoxify the body.

Additionally, if you eat saturated fats such as meats, ghee or coconut oil, it's better to drink warm water. Traditional sciences believe that cold drinks and water can make the fat congeal within the body. In fact, in both Ayurveda and TCM, water and your meals must be well spaced—at least

30-45 minutes before and after meals—so as to not dilute the nutrients of food. You can drink maybe a cup with food, but no more.

Water that is charged with electrolytes such as sodium and potassium tends to hydrate the body better. The simple practice of adding a few sprigs of mint, lemongrass or a slice or two of cucumber or orange enhances the taste, increases the electrolyte content and makes it easier to drink. An ancient practice is to also use containers in various materials to infuse the water.

✿ Copper

It is an old Indian practice to drink water from a copper tumbler. I like to infuse this water, also called *tamra jal*, overnight for at least 8 hours and drink from it upon waking up. This was suggested by my ayurvedic doctor, who explained that copper water increases the peristaltic movement of the intestines over the course of two-three months, which ultimately improves digestion. Copper water is also naturally antibacterial, improves thyroid health and balances all three doshas of the body.

Recent studies have shown that drinking water stored in a copper container kills bacteria such as salmonella and E. Coli. It also alkalizes it by slightly increasing the pH. In the study water, was stored for 16 hours for the pH to change. With this in mind, store water for at least 12 hours, if not more, to get maximum benefits from this ancient metal.

✿ Clay + vetiver

Most of us have grown up with the familiarity of water from earthen *matkas*. The perfectly cool temperature and slightly earthy flavour make this more delicious than refrigerated water. It is believed that storing water in a terracotta *surahi* or matka makes it more alkaline and mineral rich. In Ayurveda, it is also believed that meats are best cooked in clay pots because the alkalinity of the terracotta takes away the acidity from animal fat. Perhaps this is reason why in the old days an earthen pot was used to boil milk and store dairy products such as butter and yoghurt.

You can further enhance the earthy taste of the matka by adding a small ball of whole vetiver root. Also known as khus, this medicinal grass is antiseptic, anti-inflammatory, and particularly works to calm the nervous and circulatory systems. If you want to add vetiver root to a matka of water, it must be no more than the size of a golf ball. If you want to add it to your water bottle, then it must be much less. In excessive quantities vetiver can make the water bitter, so a little goes a long way.

4

FASTING AND DETOXIFICATION

Fasting is a huge component of meditation retreats. At a Zen retreat that I visited in southern Japan, we followed the Nishi Health protocol where we fasted for 18 hours every day. Dinner was at 5 p.m. and the first meal was lunch the next day, between 12 and 1 p.m. A ten-day vipassana course is even more challenging. The last meal is at 11 a.m., though newbies like me were allowed a cup of chai and a portion of puffed rice around 5 p.m. I think it's easier to be disciplined about food at a retreat that is based on frugality. But fasting in everyday life can be challenging, even though it is certainly beneficial, given our overconsumption in the city.

Indian fasts of course are quite different and perhaps can't come under the modern fasting protocol. Even on a day when one meal is allowed, we eat yoghurt, bananas, sweets, *sabudana* khichri, *kuttu* rotis, potato cutlets and halwa. Of course, during Navratri, we also have *vrat thalis* (oh, the irony), which defy all basic tenets of fasting.

Every religion has a fasting tradition, be it Ramadan or Lent in Christianity. Putting fasting within the context of

spirituality gives it mass appeal and makes it easier to adopt. Even though the practice may have had its origins in health and wellness, over the years, the concept has become distorted. We now fast purely for religious purposes, having completely forgotten its health benefits. Thankfully, new data brings this practice back into focus across the world. Considered to be the magic elixir of well-being, fasting is seeing a revival, and the best part is that it comes without religious undertones.

Modern Revival

When we abstain from food, we give our internal organs (which otherwise go through a constant cycle of digestion, assimilation and detoxification) a break. Studies have proved that the body begins the process of autophagy after 12 hours of no food. This means that when starved, your body begins to feed on its cells. It sounds morbid, but here's the good part: the first cells to go in the process are the unnecessary or diseased cell components, and therefore, this is the body's most natural method of detoxification.

Studies have found that those who fasted for more than 13 hours had lower chances of breast cancer. It was also found that intermittent fasting reduces inflammation, enhances metabolism, clears toxins from damaged cells and improves a range of ailments. But while many follow the 16:8 protocol of fasting 16 hours and eating only in the 8-hour window, it works even better when done in harmony with the circadian rhythm, i.e., between 7 a.m. and 5-6 p.m.

The research on this subject is certainly new, but the concept itself is very old. Indians traditionally have always

fasted intermittently. The concept of *do waqt ki roti* was about two meals in a day—one after sunrise and the other before sunset. But fasting isn't just a part of Indian tradition—many physicians and philosophers have waxed lyrical about its powerful effects. Rumi said that 'Fasting is the first principle of medicine; fast and see the strength of the spirit reveal itself.' Benjamin Franklin famously said, 'The best of all medicine is resting and fasting.' The fact is that fasting is resting for our internal organs. Even while we sleep, our body is constantly working to process food, detoxify the cells, rebuild tissue. By taking a break from food, we are giving the body an opportunity to heal itself.

The Traditional View

Every culture and religion has a tradition of fasting. Moses fasted for 120 days, Jesus for forty days. Ramadan is a yearly month-long fast based on the lunar cycles. The Hindu *ekadashi* fast is also observed with the lunar cycle (every eleventh day after the full moon). Many believe—even though there isn't any conclusive evidence—that during certain days (full or new moon, ekadashi) of the months, the moon affects the atmospheric pressure on the earth, which makes these days better for detoxifying the body. *Upvasa*, the Sanskrit word for fasting, means to 'stay near the almighty'. Ayurvedic texts say, '*langham param aushadham*', meaning fasting is the greatest medicine. The practice of abstinence is said to purify the body, strengthen the mind and help connect with the higher consciousness.

A spiritual/religious reason to abstain from food gives motivation to some. Or you could get your motivation from the research that supports this incredible practice.

The Right Way to Fast

1) Eat Right

In the modern-day practice of intermittent fasting, many see the 8-hour window to eat as a free pass to indulge in comfort food. But for this practice to be effective, even during the periods one isn't fasting, food must be eaten in moderation and should help build the body and not break it down. Choose whole foods, fruit and vegetable, clean sources of protein, lean meats and healthy, unrefined fats.

Doctors and nutritionists warn about the binge/fast cycle. When you consume food with trans fats, refined carbohydrates and sugars, your body has to work doubly hard to process these ingredients. Because heavy food takes longer to digest, you're utilizing energy that could have otherwise been used to detoxify the body at a cellular level. Detoxification is the body's last priority, as active functions such as movement and digestion take precedence. Therefore, even if you fast for shorter periods, fast completely. Even a morsel of food, will shift the focus from the body's function of purification to digestion.

Of course, it is absolutely necessary to enjoy your favourite foods occasionally, but treat them as a weekly treat. As you continue to eat whole, fresh food and fast minimally, you will see the effects of this traditional practice. It isn't about weight loss—fasting gives a boost

of energy, a feeling of lightness and clarity of thought. Personally, I find it difficult to fast because of my vata-dominant constitution, prone to fatigue and lower weight. I usually follow a 12-hour fast. If longer fasts suit your constitution, only then they can be sustained.

2) Follow the Circadian Rhythms

Intermittent fasting may give you an excuse to eat your last meal at 10 p.m. and first meal at 2 p.m., but recent studies have shown that it works best when practised in line with circadian rhythms or with the day and night cycle. Also called time restricted feeding (TRF), where you eat for eight to ten hours during the hours of sunlight, it showed reduced parameters such as lower body fat, insulin levels, inflammation and hyperlipidaemia, especially when food was concentrated during midday. Eating later around the afternoon or evening seemed to either nullify or worsen glucose, blood pressure and lipid levels.

Whether you call it time-restricted feeding or the circadian diet, fact is that science is just proving what tradition has believed. Ayurveda recommends eating your main, heaviest meal at mid-day because that is when the *jatharagni* or digestive fire is at its peak. It is also strongly recommended that the last meal of the day must ideally be consumed around sunset. It isn't just about what you eat, but when you eat. Just shifting your meal timings will have a transformational effect, because eating at the right time means digesting at the right time, clearing the way for detoxification.

3) Rest well

Sleep is the best ally of any detox. During my panchakarma, which I found to be a fairly intensive, I found that my body was more exhausted than after a 90-minute ashtanga class. If you choose to fast a couple of days in the week, or even intermittently every day, rest must be prioritized. But even though rest is required during any extended detox, Ayurveda doesn't recommend daytime napping. Unless it's in the harsh summer months of India or you're over the age of sixty, daytime naps increase the production of *ama* or toxins in the body, which is counterproductive to fasting. According to Ayurveda, daytime naps increase *kapha* (weight gain) and *pitta* (inflammation). Because naps increase toxicity— including conditions such as migraines, obesity, colds, cough and congestion, among others—they're especially not recommended during spring, when kapha increases naturally in the body. If one really has to nap, do so sitting comfortably so that the torso remains upright, instead of lying down.

4) Listen to your Body

The modern age makes a fetish out of traditional practices. In its enthusiasm to promote these rituals as one-stop cures, we gloss over the details. Within the realm of fasting, even though it has myriad benefits, the concept of fasting daily for 16-18 hours could be extreme, especially if you have a very active daily routine. Many practitioners complain about constipation as one side effect and fatigue as another. It is important to note that in every tradition, fasting is

never recommended as a continuous practice. Whether its Ramadan, Ekadashi or Lent, fasting is recommended for limited periods of time. It's always a good idea to consult a health professional if you have health conditions or if fasting doesn't suit you.

5) Fast from Stimulation

Fasting isn't limited to just food, since we consume from all senses. Detoxification from other sources of stimulation also falls under the aegis of fasting. Taking a break from social media, excessive conversation or anxiety-inducing content give hyper-stimulated sense organs a rest. Because the concept of fasting isn't limited to purification; it is also meant to reduce extreme attachments. Fasting from food is just the beginning. As you see its benefits, try applying it to other aspects of life (where you have an unhealthy attachment) for limited periods to feel lighter and more refreshed.

6) Breaking the Fast

Though it may be tempting to indulge in your favourite dessert after fasting, it's important to choose the healthiest options that won't cause blood sugar to rise. This means non-starchy vegetables, healthy fats, seeds, nuts, fruit like apples and berries that aren't very sweet, plus proteins such as fish, poultry or beans. Think of your body like a fresh canvas—introduce only the healthiest, most nourishing foods on this clean slate. Keep your treats for later after you've 'lined' the stomach with healthy food.

What is right for you?

There are many ways to give your internal organs a break. You could fast on the daily for 12–13 hours. You could choose one day in the week where you eat only one meal in the day, choosing fruit and vegetable for the remainder of the time. Or, if you're experienced and have practised it under the tutelage of a doctor or guru, you could drink only water for a day. Personally, my vata-dominant constitution demands food. I eat dinner around 8 p.m. and breakfast between 8 a.m. to 9 a.m., so I take a 12–13 hour break on a daily basis. Taking a break from sugar, dairy, grains and meat would qualify as a fast as well, since these ingredients are hard to metabolize and cause inflammation. Moderation and curation must be practised before ritualizing daily routines. What suits me may not suit you and vice versa, and that is especially true of fasting.

A lot has been said about fasting, its connection with autophagy and the effect on cancer cells. Certainly, autophagy does have an effect, however, it depends on the tissue. For instance, when it comes to the breast, it definitely shows positive effects; however, food restrictions could also increase problems in the heart. There are animal studies to show that not only fasting, but also curcumin and exercise also lead to autophagy. The point is that anything is bad when practised in excess. Not everything that is trending will work for you. So, listen to your body, learn to read its signals and practise moderation for steady, long-term health benefits.

PILLAR II

✳

Energize

> Where there is pain there is no movement,
> where there is movement there is no pain.
>
> —Huang Di Nei Jing

In TCM, movement, or obstruction-free flow of energy, leads to prevention of illness. Energy, known as qi in the TCM and prana in yoga, is the essential life force that resides within all living beings. Just like prana has many different variations in Ayurveda, qi too has several applications. The qi of the food is good when it tastes pleasant and provides nutrition. A person who has physical strength has 'abundant' qi, whereas someone with a sharp, clear mind has 'refined' qi. Conversely, if someone does not have clarity of thought, they have 'confused' qi. This word in Chinese medicine is an accurate measure of the level and type of vitality in every object—animate or inanimate.

In Hindu mythology, energy is defined as Shakti, without which Shiva would only be consciousness without creation. There are in fact five powers within Shakti written about in the Shiva Sutras. All of us have access to these powers, namely *chitta shakti, jnana shakti, kriya shakti, iccha shakti* and *ananda shakti.* Chitta shakti, or the power of consciousness, means to tap into the part of your mind unsullied by knowledge or

experience. Then there are jnana and kriya shakti—like the names suggest, they come from knowledge and the ability to act. Iccha shakti is born out of the force of will. Lastly, there is ananda shakti, to be in touch with pure consciousness for the purpose of bliss. As we know through experience, bliss is the best kind of energy out of them all. And even though bliss may sound elusive, it can be found in small moments such as sitting down after a long run or the refreshing taste of water when you're thoroughly parched.

In physics, the law of conservation of energy states that energy isn't created or destroyed but converted from one form to another, or transferred from one object to another. This means that an object will always have a similar amount of energy, unless it is added from the outside. A simple example would be soccer, where the energy from your foot is transferred to the ball. A more esoteric concept would be how we feel elevated or depleted depending on optimism or pessimism, absorbed via people or circumstances. Within the framework of health and wellness, this concept is apparent in diet—a light, nutritious diet uplifts as compared to heavy, greasy food that makes you feel leaden.

'Strength doesn't come from physical capacity. It comes from an indomitable will,' said Mahatma Gandhi. This quote perfectly illustrates the concept of mental energy. Today, this phrase is backed by scientific studies. The most popular example is the marshmallow test, where sweets were placed in front of toddlers. If they could wait for the researcher to come back, they would get two, if not, they would get one. Thirty years later, when followed up, it was found that the children who waited for the candy scored better on their SATs and

had a lower body mass index (BMI). Undoubtedly, the building blocks of any type of success—monetary, creative or spiritual—are patience, willpower and self-control. To cultivate these attributes, we require mental energy.

Like all good things in life, vitality isn't built in a day, but results from consistency. Whether via pranayama, exercise or healthy food, we need to be invigorated several times a day, because we also expend energy every few hours. Even the flow of this energy needs to be maintained so there are no blockages. All traditional sciences (be it Ayurveda or TCM) believe that disease always begins with blockage/stagnation of energy. For instance, according to Ayurveda, endometriosis happens because there is a blockage in the *apana vayu*, or the downward flow of energy. In TCM stress and anxiety are the primary causes that lead to stagnant qi, which is reflected in depression, anger, mood swings, painful periods and can lead to chronic disease.

As energy ebbs and flows through the day, this pillar of the sun requires a layered approach. To be truly refreshed, we need to be physically, mentally and spiritually energized. The following chapters detail elements that give you a boost, both long and short-term. You can choose between a quick rush when you feel most depleted, or practices that build reserves over the long term. For me, certain pranayamas practised in the morning work to clarify thoughts and increase vitality. For you, it could be a mid-afternoon snack that boosts productivity. It is entirely up to you to pick and choose rituals that work with your interests and schedule.

Ultimately, it is not possible to utilize this entire arsenal of practices. While the rules of food and drink must be

imbibed, in terms of yogic remedies, begin by choosing just one. Chinese medicine practitioners say you cannot wear too many hats at the same time. Therefore, don't load up with too many practices in an already-packed schedule. Start with one, and add another only after you're habituated to the first. Too many hats make the head heavy, so keep it light and take your time, so that you're consistent. Rituals require a lifetime of refinement, so layer one after the other till you find your comfortable space.

1

SUNBATHING

One of the most important principles of Ayurveda is the *pindi* to *brahmandi* concept. The human body, the *pind* or microcosm, is considered to be the mirror or miniature of the universe, the bramhandi or macrocosm. Just like there is heat and energy in the stars, heat and energy are present in our bodies too. And if we look at anatomy as not just the physical body but also the emotions and auric field, exposing ourselves to the elements helps balance body and mind, especially today when technology takes us away our true nature. Whether it's grounding the feet on grass wet with dew drops to calm anxiety, dipping them in sea water to cleanse negativity or sunbathing to boost the mood and energy, going to back to nature means healing ourselves from the inside out.

We know that the sun helps with wakefulness, energy and clarity. Decisions made during the night are clearer in daylight. The sun is responsible for stimulating several hormones associated with these responses. Just like melatonin is responsible for the inertia of nighttime, serotonin is the

by-product of sunshine. It has been found that serotonin, also known as the happy hormone, gets a boost with daylight and sunshine. In fact, it can be produced by our skin because both serotonin and its transporters have been found in keratinocytes, cells that make up 90 per cent of the epidermis. Though these findings are preliminary, there is evidence that sunshine has a role in the production of this feel-good hormone. Perhaps this is the reason why anything from minutes to hours of warm sun helps elevate our mood and feeling of comfort.

In the current scenario, sunbathing has rightfully earned itself a poor reputation because it's usually done between 11 a.m. and 4 p.m., when sunrays are most powerful. But I'm talking about is sunbathing for a very short time, in the morning or evening, when the rays are gentlest. Part of traditional yogic practices, this form of sun worship removes disease-causing pathogens, invigorates muscles and tissues, and clears and energizes the mind. I visited Kerala earlier this year and learnt a Malayalam saying that encapsulates traditional beliefs in solar power, '*Andhi vela konda chanda tamra pole agam.*' This means that if you catch the last rays of the sun, you'll bloom like the red lotus. This is more in the context of sun-gazing.

There are many yogis in India who regularly practise sun-gazing, with some who live off the energy provided by the sun, with limited portions of food. But these are enlightened beings, who have every aspect of their life streamlined with this practice. Despite its benefits, sun-gazing isn't enough to sustain most humans, especially those who live a high-

stress life. However, heliotherapy or sunbathing for holistic purposes can be practised by one and all.

Safe Sunbathing

Traditionally, sunbaths were taken first thing in the morning, when the sun's rays are gentlest. The morning sun is healing, whether you gaze at its diffused light or bathe under its subtle rays. The ideal daily sunlight exposure for effective synthesis of vitamin D is when 20 per cent of the body is exposed to the sun for 30 minutes, if you're at sea level. For people who work indoors most of the day, it is recommended that they utilize an hour during the weekend for safe sun exposure. A secure time to harness the sun's immense healing potential is early morning, typically before 8 a.m. and after 5 p.m. In winter, you can enjoy the soft sunshine for up to half an hour, but in the warmer months, it must be limited to 10-15 minutes every day.

When practised wisely, there isn't any reason to be afraid of sunlight. Stay in the sun only till you can tolerate it, not a minute longer. Apply an oil such as sesame before your morning sunbath for better penetration and blood circulation. Take a bath afterwards; do not eat immediately but after half hour or so.

2

BREATHWORK

Breathing is the most automatic yet versatile function of the body. Even though it happens naturally, when you learn to control and channelize it, it can be used to relax, energize, heal or increase concentration. How you breathe indicates the state of your physical and mental condition. When we're stressed, our breath is shallow, therefore to relax, we inhale deeply. Breathing is such a natural process that it's easy to disconnect from it completely. However, the breath is the bridge between the mind and the body. Whenever you find your mind slipping away, bring your attention to each inhale and exhale to unify mind and body.

In yoga, the correct sequence for advancement is asana, then pranayama, and finally meditation. However, in this day and age, the focus is primarily on asana and meditation. But meditation itself can be dangerous if not practised under the tutelage of an experienced teacher. If your mind is not in your control, sitting in silence could weigh you down with thoughts. Pranayama, on the other hand, is much safer. The

deep, conscious inhales and exhales help release heaviness, relax the mind, energise and oxygenate the body.

Studies have proved that pranayama enhances cognitive function, reduces stress and strengthens lungs, thereby improving immunity. Yogis are known to have studied animals, whether it's for yoga poses or breathing practices. Through this observation, they realized that animals that breathe slowly have longer lifespans than those with shorter, shallow breaths. For instance, a tortoise takes 4 breaths a minute and lives up to 120 years, whereas a dog breathes an average of 24 breaths per minute and is expected to live between twelve and fifteen years. In this sense, slow breathing seems to extend lifespan.

Breathwork isn't just good for long-terms benefits but also provides instant gratification. A few deep inhales instantly make you feel better. In just a few minutes, pranayama can make you feel calm when you're agitated, or focused when your thoughts are scattered. People recommend meditation to reduce stress, but a few minutes of pranayama before meditation helps centre the mind and therefore refine your meditative practice. But pranayama strands as a practice on its own, with or without asana or meditation. In a world where focus and patience are anomalies, it is more realistic (and doable) to just breathe.

An exercise for when you're stressed: breathe deeply, feeling your breath enter your nostrils, tracing its path down your throat, to the chest, down the stomach, all the way to the pelvic floor. And now follow the path of the breath in the same way while you exhale. Take 25 deep breaths in this manner.

Making Friends with your Breath

Set a timer for 2–5 minutes. Lie down in bed and focus on your breath. Do not change it in any manner. If it's shallow, let it be. If it's deep, accept it as it is. Just trace its movements, observe which nostril is more open, become aware of its sensations, whether they're warm or cool. If the mind runs, which it will, bring it back to the present moment, without any agitation, repeatedly, till the time is up. We go out into the world to seek knowledge but most of us aren't even aware of how we breathe.

Surya Bhedana

If you like to dive into activity upon waking up, it may serve you well to practise right nostril breathing for a few minutes. The practice of inhaling through a single nostril can have either an activating or a relaxing effect. Inhaling via the right nostril is called *surya bhedana*, literally translated into 'sun

piercing' breath. I have found this pranayama to be especially beneficial first thing in the morning.

- ✿ Close your left nostril with your left thumb and inhale through the right nostril to activate the surya nadi.
- ✿ Then close the right nostril with your left ring finger and exhale through the left.
- ✿ Repeat by inhaling through the right nostril and exhaling through the left.
- ✿ Please note that surya bhedana must not be practised by those with high blood pressure or in the very hot months of summer.

Did you know?

Focusing on the inhale activates the alert modes. Therefore, concentrate on your inhales during breathwork in the morning to feel fresher and keep the mind sharper.

Nadi Shodhana

Some years ago, I attended Dr Robert Svoboda's talk on tantra. During the lecture, he said that if there was just one spiritual practice to be continued for the rest of your life, choose alternate nostril breathing. Also known as *anulom vilom*, this is perhaps the most popular pranayama, with good reason. It requires no special expertise, spiritual advancement

or physical strength—the only thing that it requires is patience. It's precisely this simplicity that makes it such a special practice, which boosts energy, calms the nervous system, enhances immunity and provides mental clarity.

To understand how this exercise works, we need to delve into the ethereal network of channels which pass through the body, infusing it with energy and vitality. Called meridians in Chinese medicine and nadis in Ayurveda, these pathways are responsible for the smooth flow of prana, qi or the essential life force. Out of the 72,000 nadis in the body, the most important are the ida (left nostril) and pingala (right nostril). The left is ruled by the moon and is feminine, creative and emotional, while the right ruled by the sun, is masculine, physical and practical. This pranayama is also known as *nadi shodhana* because it helps purify these channels and balances the two opposites of the sun and moon aspects of our physiology and personality.

Ayurvedic practitioners believe that disease begins when the flow of prana gets obstructed. Think about how your breath changes when you're under stress. The breath becomes shallow, and depending on your personal body type, you may feel an obstruction a blockage, be it a lump in your throat, a knot in your chest or a brick in your stomach. There is no doubt that most diseases begin in the mind. Stress causes the body to spin out of balance, eventually causing disease. The bridge in between the body and the mind is the breath.

While it is challenging to change circumstances in an instant, at the very least, we can use the breath to release heaviness in the body and thereby calm the mind. With pranayama, the change is almost instantaneous, though

temporary in the short term. Even though you may step back into the stressful situation, during those moments of deep breathing, it is possible to find some fleeting peace. Sometimes, just a few moments of tranquillity are enough.

How to Practice Nadi Shodhana

✿ Sit in a comfortable position with your back straight. You can sit either cross-legged or on a chair with both feet flat on the floor. Keep the chin tucked in slightly—think of the action as straightening the back of your neck, or that you're pushing the head back so the chin tucks in. Do not let your chest cave inwards, keep your torso lifted and back upright so that energy can flow easily in a straight spine. If required, place a small cushion behind your lower back to keep the spine from curving.

✿ If you're right-handed, place your thumb gently on your right nostril and ring finger on your left nostril. Start by gently pressing the right nostril and inhaling through the left. Close both nostrils for a second then exhale though the right. Then inhale through the right and exhale through the left. One inhale and exhale from both nostrils completes one set. Try to do at least ten sets.

✿ Don't use inhale sharply and don't throw your breath out with the exhale. Keep your breath so soft that you're unable to hear it.

✿ Trail the movement of your breath as you inhale and exhale. I like to imagine both nadis in a 'U' shape. When my breath touches the base of the 'U', I hold my breath for a few seconds and then exhale. Don't attempt

retention when you begin. The breath must be tamed slowly, otherwise it can cause adverse effects. It better to stick to simpler practices—advanced variations must be learnt from a teacher.

☼ If your hand gets tired, change the hand when you hold the breath.

☼ It is natural that you will engage with several thoughts, you might also get irritated or agitated. Don't berate yourself when that happens, just bring your attention back to your breath without the feeling of frustration.

☼ After pranayama, lie down flat in shavasana for 2 minutes so that the body can reap the benefits.

Three-Part Breathing

Pranayama is energizing for the body and calming for the mind. However, one of its lesser talked about benefits is detoxification. Our lymph nodes are also situated below the diaphragm. Because of this, deep breathing that pushes and opens the diaphragm helps in stimulating the movement of lymph, leading to detoxification. Three-part breathing, where you first breathe into the pelvic floor followed by the stomach and lungs is calming, grounding and detoxifying.

Most pranayama is best done slowly and this one is no different. As your breath slows, it centres and relaxes the mind which results in better focus before you begin the day. If you have the time you can practice this three-part breath prior to the alternate nostril breathing, or choose only to do just this if the finger movements for anulom vilom are tiring or distracting:

○ Sit in a comfortable position with your back straight. Keeping your eyes closed, breathe in, directing the breath into your pelvic floor and filling up your lower abdomen. Your belly must expand with the breath. Do three rounds of lower abdomen breathing.

○ Then breath into your upper stomach, pushing it outwards. As you inhale, the diaphragm pushes downward, so really feel this downward push as you inhale. Do three rounds.

○ Finally, fill your lower abdomen, stomach and lungs till the throat. As you do this, imagine the breath filling up the front, back and sides of the lungs. You'll be surprised to know that most of our lungs are situated in the back (not front) of the body.

○ Exhale slowly, letting the air out first from the throat, then lungs, followed by the stomach, feeling your diaphragm go up as you release. I like to sometimes focus just on the diaphragm—it's fascinating how it goes down on the inhale and lifts up when you breathe out. Finally, exhale from your belly button and pelvis. Practise 3 to 5 rounds.

3

MOVEMENT

It's interesting that as we age, we see a decrease in both movement and energy in our body. It's a vicious cycle—the less energized we feel the more opposed we are to any sort of movement. But even the minutest motions of the body keep it supple, preventing degradation. Think about how the fingers are exercised with activities such as sports, crafts and writing letters. Or how the muscle is built up in weight training and how that strengthens the core. Observe how yoga stretches the ligaments, tones muscles and opens tight joints. Even a simple activity like walking keeps the body and mind light.

Whatever may be your choice of movement, they provide that undeniable rush of energy and boost of endorphins. But exercise can be intimidating, especially in the world of social media, where everything is in hyperbole, it is seen as effective only when it is in the extreme. But every fitness expert will tell you to choose consistency over intensity. Even beginning with a 15-minute daily walk is a good start. It's only natural that as you become more consistent, you'll become motivated take it up another level. Small, consistent workouts are also

a safer way to exercise. I've injured my IT band, sprained my hamstrings and my shoulders only to contort my body into a pose that wasn't suitable for me. The ego boost in lifting more or powering through a longer run is undeniably addictive and beneficial in competitive sports. But when the ego is in charge in personal practice it leads to injuries. Think about the time when you ran that extra kilometre when people were watching or the arm balance that you lifted into during yoga class. While there is no doubt we must push ourselves, we must be cognizant of the body's boundaries.

Seema Sondhi, my yoga guru, always says, 'You're not going to get a gold medal in your yoga practice.' And yet we exercise like there is a trophy waiting for us towards the end. Not everyone can exercise hard, run for miles or hold an arm balance. And that's okay. The moment I removed the idea of competition from my workouts, I started healing. Some of the best exercises are low intensity, like walking. It doesn't matter how hard your workout may be—what works is to be consistent, at least five to six days a week.

Studies have shown us that 30 minutes of cardio four days a week is enough to stay healthy. We make it complicated by making workout plans so exhaustive that they're impossible to follow on a daily basis. The right exercise plans must a) fit into your schedule and b) should energize you instead of wearing you out. The best exercise can also be as simple as a brisk walk.

During the times of COVID-19, I enthusiastically chose brisk walking as my primary form of exercise. Being generally injury-prone, it was a mini workout but with very little chance of a strain. Walking enhances cardiovascular health, lowers BMI, and is even known to improve memory and cognitive

function. Even though the right exercise should be a mix of functional training, resistance work, flexibility and weights, walking for 30 minutes once or twice a day is enough to live a healthful life.

There are many things you can combine with walking to double the benefits. You can recite a mantra or affirmation, focus on your breath, listen to great music or just observe everything around you. Unlike other workouts that demand undivided attention, walking, yoga or cycling or any self-practice is a great way to introspect. My gynaecologist recommends walking and running for women who have issues such as endometriosis and PCOD. While running too is a natural function of the body, it takes time to build stamina and some guidance to ensure you don't injure your back or knees.

Though eventually it's a good idea to push yourself to build greater levels of strength, flexibility and endurance, movement must always be enjoyed. Think about how we moved as children. We ran, played and jumped because it was fun. So, look beyond yoga, gym, walking or pilates. Some people love to clean, others love to dance. I discovered with my niece that I loved jumping on the trampoline. Either way, if you have just 10 minutes in the morning, move your body for that instant boost of in mood and energy. It will take a bit of adjusting to it if you're new, but once it becomes a habit, you'll do happily.

The Five Tibetan Rites

More than 2,500 years old, these rites, practiced by Tibetan lamas, help balance chakras, keep the joints supple and

body strong, and provide spiritual benefits. Because they are practiced by the Tibetan lamas, these must be practised by those who are already fit and have good core strength. It's a good sequence to fit in on days when you want the simplicity and intensity at the same time.

I first heard about these rites from a sanyasi at a panchakarma centre in Pune. Each 'rite' is an exercise that needs to be repeated 21 times. Also called the 'fountain of youth', these exercises, it is believed, balance the energy vortexes in the body and boost energy. The Tibetans believe that we have seven main energy vortexes or chakras, which spin at a great speed. The main cause of ageing and ailments is the slowing down of these chakras.

These five exercises restore the normal functioning of the chakras, and therefore are referred to as rites instead of exercises because they go beyond just the physical body. Though each rite is practised in sets of twenty-one reps., do not attempt the required number of reps right away. Start with three, five, seven and nine and build it up in odd numbers, which the Tibetans believe are auspicious. Never practise more than the required twenty-one reps as that may have adverse effects.

Also remember that the speed of number of reps doesn't matter. What matters more is how you coordinate the movement with your breath. When we focus on our inhale and exhale, the movement has psycho-spiritual benefits, as opposed to pushing ourselves beyond limits that leads to an injured body and an agitated mind. If you're out of breath, stop right away. Eventually, you will have enough stamina to do all the reps harmoniously with the breath.

I love these exercises because they can be done in the comfort of your home, for the rest of your life. The whole ritual takes 10 minutes only and builds you up so that you will have strong bones and flexible joints in old age. It's also perfect for the morning, because it gives that boost of energy.

1. Rite no. 1

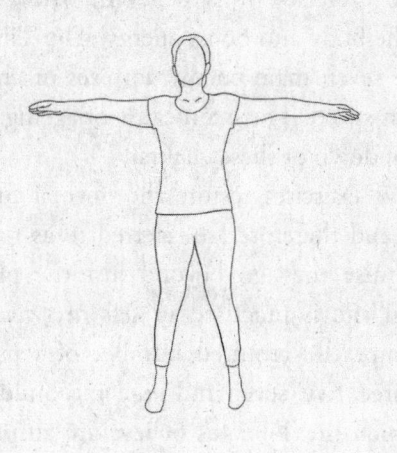

Rite 1

Start by spreading your arms out, then start spinning in a clockwise direction, keeping your eyes open, and gaze downwards towards the floor. This will make you dizzy when you begin, so it's wise to start with a smaller number of reps and then build up. (Do not practice this if you have vertigo.) Lie down and rest for a few seconds before you begin the next pose.

2. Rite no. 2

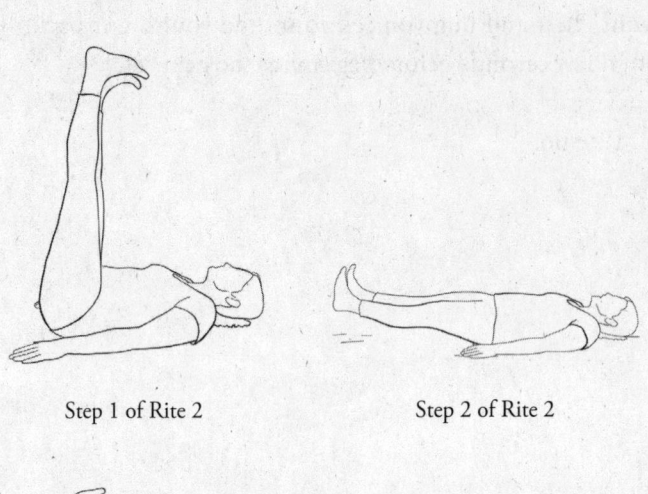

Step 1 of Rite 2   Step 2 of Rite 2

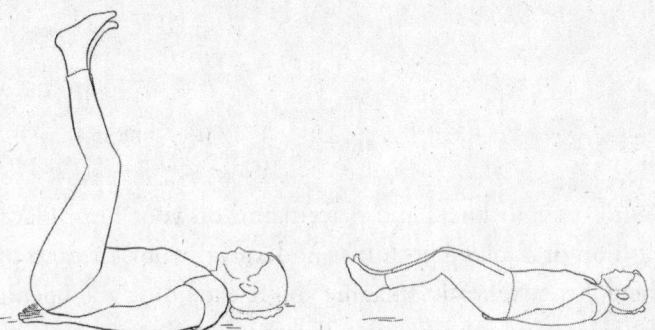

Gentle variation of Step 1 of Rite 2   Gentle variation of Step 2 of Rite 2

Lie down on a mat. Then keeping your spine straight, both shoulders on the mat and chin slightly tucked in, raise both legs straight till they're at a right angle with your body and then bring them down. If you have a weak or injured back, keep your knees gently bent and place your palms (face

down) to support your lower back. Start small and then build up your strength. Once you finish, bring your knees close to your chest and hug yourself to soothe your lower back. Rest for a few seconds before beginning the next set.

3. Rite no. 3

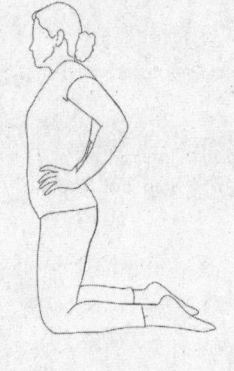 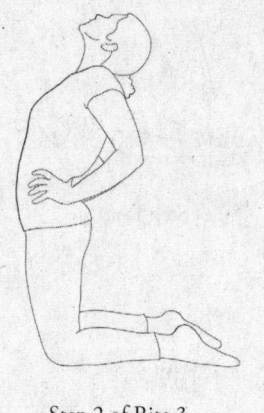

Step 1 of Rite 3   Step 2 of Rite 3

Stand on your knees and place palms on your hips. Place a cushion or a folded yoga mat underneath your knees to pad them if they're weak) Imagine you're extending and opening the front of your body—first lengthen the front of the pelvis, opening the belly, rolling your shoulders back and open the chest and then bend backwards gently. Keep in mind that you must focus on opening and lengthening the front part of the body. Do not bend backwards from your lower back as that will compress your spine—focus more on opening the chest.

Keep the gaze at the chest, at the ceiling or (if you're very open) look back. Come back to neutral position and repeat no more than 21 times. Don't forget to relax for a few seconds before you get into the next pose.

4. Rite no. 4

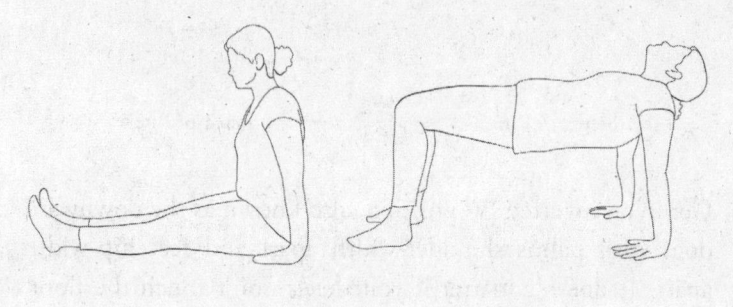

Step 1 of Rite 4   Step 2 of Rite 4

Sit with your legs stretched in front of you and palms on the side of your hips. From position swing your hips upwards till you reach a 'tabletop' position where your legs are bent at a 90-degree angle, body straight opening upwards, and palms grounded and feet planted on the floor. Hold for 1 second and then sit back in the same position. Eventually, work up to 21 reps. Make sure you keep your stomach gently pulled in to protect your back.

5. Rite no.5

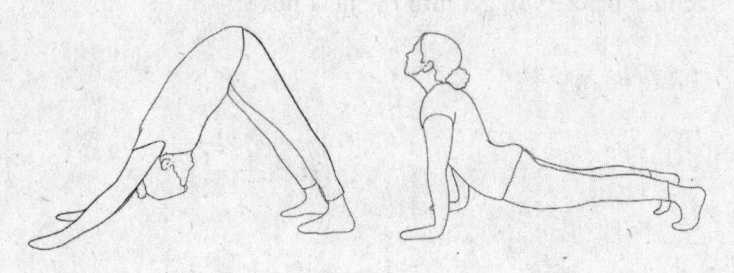

Step 2 of Rite 5   Step 1 of Rite 5

Get in an inverted 'V' position, also known as the downward dog, with palms shoulder-width apart and feet hip-width apart. It doesn't matter if your heels don't touch the floor. From here, move forward, keeping your toes tucked in, knees and hips off the floor. Open your chest and shoulders, and (if it doesn't strain your neck) look up. Then go back into the downward. Repeat no more than 21 times.

4

AFTERNOON BOOSTERS

For someone who enjoys writing from the comfort of her own home, I find my productivity dipping to the lowest during the afternoons. Of course, one should never work from the comfort of their couch. That is a bad habit I need to get rid of right after I finish this book. But even if you don't work from home, being productive after lunch takes an immense amount of determination. Here's a reality check to help keep you awake during the day: daytime naps are not recommended in Ayurveda. It is believed that lying down for a nap after lunch is a sure-fire way to increase ama or toxins within the body. In fact, during panchakarma, naps are strictly forbidden since it increases the toxins that you are trying to eliminate. The only exceptions—during high summer or if you're over sixty-five.

Non-Sleep Deep Rest (NDSR)

Rest is possible even when the mind is awake. Guided meditations that require us to shift our thoughts help relax

and recuperate. *Yoga nidra*, a guided meditation, is now a fairly popular practice, which I turn to, especially when I know that I have to rest but may be unable to fall asleep. Or when I wake up in the middle of the night, I prefer to practise this instead of going through my phone. There are many types of yoga nidra available with a quick search on the phone. I like to choose a longer one when I know I need to sleep and a shorter one when I need a pick-up during the afternoon. Because yoga nidra completely relaxes the nervous system, it is believed that it helps us connect with our subconscious. Therefore, a *sankalpa* or positive affirmation is to be repeated 3 times with full belief before and after the practice. I like to keep only one sankalpa for this meditation, something that I would like to work towards in this life. Ideally, one should stay awake during this practice; however, if one needs to sleep, or even relax, then one should let go and allow the body to rest, for a short while.

Simple Chair Stretches

Sometimes, simplicity can complicate lives even though it will eventually bring about a transformation. Like the most elementary health habit of following the circadian rhythms— if you wake up around sunrise and sleep around 10 p.m., you will most definitely stay in good health and won't require detoxes, superfoods or supplements. Synchronizing your routine according to the rise and fall of the sun makes your body function optimally because every hour in the day belongs to the function of a separate organ. By eating, sleeping and exercising according to nature's cycle, you keep your internal

engineering functioning optimally. But it's easier said than done. In the earlier days when our schedules were similar as a collective, this was possible. Today following circadian rhythms is a privilege, because it requires a combination of the right circumstances and discipline.

The second simple change is posture. This is something I've struggled with for the majority of my life, and it's still a work in progress. The right posture ensures bone, muscle, digestive health and also prevents fatigue. Hunching compresses the internal organs and adds unnecessary pressure on the bones. A habitually poor posture also leads to fatigue because the body isn't used to holding itself up. The yogic school of thought believes that that you are as young as your spine, because the most debilitating feature of old age isn't the white hair or wrinkles, but the hunched spine and bone changes.

One way to keep our spine young is to move it in all directions, as demonstrated in the five Tibetan rites. The other way to keep it young is to build muscle so that we can hold ourselves up and correct the posture. One must stretch the body to ensure there isn't any unnecessary pressure on a certain part, which can erode the bone. But first, what is the right posture?

Simply put, the right posture while standing means to keep the weight mostly on the balls of the feet and extend the spine. Stack every part neatly one on top of another. This means that the ankles, knees, pelvis, chest, neck and head must all be in a single line, while still maintaining the natural curves on the neck and spine without any protrusions. Your pelvis would neither be pushing forward nor curved

towards the back. The chest must be open with the back of the thoracic spine pushing inwards. It is essential to check the body for any compressions. Those who have an overly arched spine will have compressions at the back, while those who are hunched will have compressions in the front of their body. The idea is to be mindful of this stacking and prevent compressions. Posture isn't something that can be corrected in day—it needs moment-to-moment awareness to keep your joints neatly stacked and the spine lengthened and lifted.

Still, as we progress in our day's work, it's common to keep the shoulders shrugged or curl deeply into our laptops. In this case, nothing works better than a few mid-afternoon chair stretches to stretch the body and refresh the mind. Keep in mind that these stretches must not be practised right after lunch but a couple of hours afterwards.

1. Restorative forward bend

Folding forward is the body's natural defence mechanism because it's restorative and calming. When you've had a day that's been completely on the go or mentally exhausting, you can find a spot of comfort with this forward fold, which can be done in two ways.

Restorative forward bend

☼ Sit on a chair and shift your hips back till they touch the backrest. Keep your feet on the floor parallel to each

other. Then, simply fold forward, allowing your head to roll between and below the knees and arms hanging straight beside you. If your chest and stomach doesn't rest on your thighs naturally, keep a cushion in between to make this pose more restorative. Stay for about a minute and lift up—you'll feel calmer and more refreshed.

✿ You can also use this pose to stretch your arms and open the chest. Fold forward in the way mentioned above, but this time, take your arms back and interlace your fingers. The difference in this variation is that your chest will be open. Remember, when you stretch your arms, they should pull back, not upwards, so that you can open the chest and create space between the shoulders and the neck.

2. The Wrist Stretch

For most of us, a day's work means hours in front of the computer tapping away at presentations. Because our wrists are mostly in one position (face down) through the day, stretching them in the opposite direction provides relief from stiffness and pain. You can simply make a fist and roll wrists in clockwise and anti-clockwise directions and try this:

✿ Stretch one arm forward, palm facing up. Hold the fingers with the opposite hand and pull them downward so you feel a stretch on the inside of your forearm. Hold for 30-60 seconds. Repeat on the other arm.

✿ Stretch one arm palm facing down. Grab hold of the fingers with the opposite hand and pull downwards so

you feel a stretch on the outer wrist. Hold for 30-60 seconds. Repeat on the other arm.

✿ Join your palms in a namaste position. Keeping your palms together in the same manner, point the fingertips downwards. You should feel a deep stretch on your wrists. Hold for the same time or shorter if it becomes unbearable.

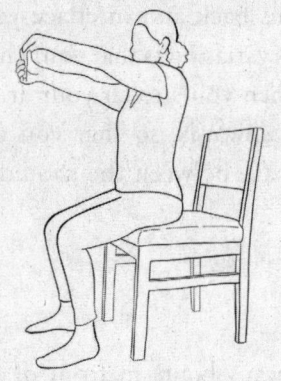
Step 1 of wrist stretch

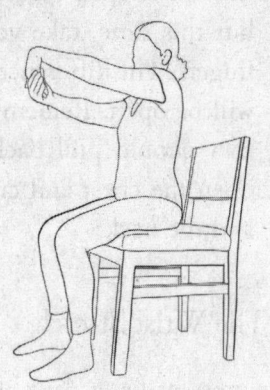
Step 2 of wrist stretch

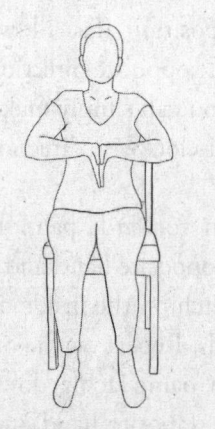
Step 3 of wrist stretch

3. The Chest Opener

No matter how mindful you may be about posture, working on the desk means hunching over. Open the chest and refresh your mind with this gentle heart opener:

Shift a little bit towards the front of your chair. Grab hold of the base of the armrests

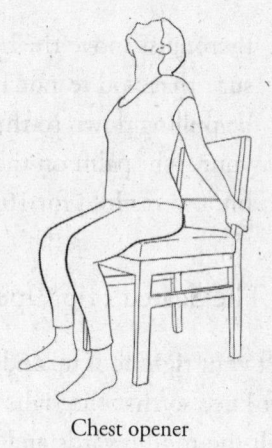

Chest opener

and stretch the front of your body, starting by pushing your hips then stomach forward and finally opening the chest and rolling the shoulders back. Look up if you want to. Do this 5-7 times. Each time, hold for a few seconds when you open the heart and roll the shoulders back.

4. The Neck Extension

This is an exercise you can even do first thing in the morning to remove any stiffness from your spine:

- ✿ Very slowly, roll your head down to the front, then to the left shoulder, back looking up, towards the right shoulder and back to the centre. Do these movements very slowly and mindfully to release any stress or tension in the neck. Do three neck rolls each in clockwise and anti-clockwise directions.
- ✿ Give your neck a side stretch by laterally rolling your head towards the right shoulder (it doesn't matter if you reach

there, just move the head towards that direction). Make sure that you're not lifting the shoulders—they should be pulling down so that there is length in the neck. Place your right palm on the right ear so the head shifts a little bit lower. Hold for 10 seconds. Repeat on the other side.

5. The Seated Hip Opener

Lift your right foot up and place the right ankle just above the left knee so that the right lower part of the leg is horizontal. Pull the toes inwards and then fold forward as much as you can. You'll feel a stretch in the right outer hip. Hold for 20-60 seconds and release. Repeat on the opposite leg.

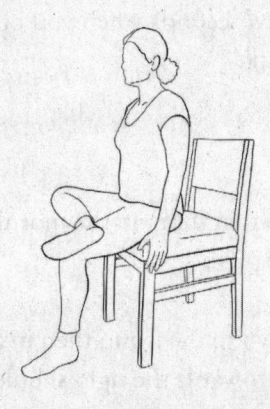
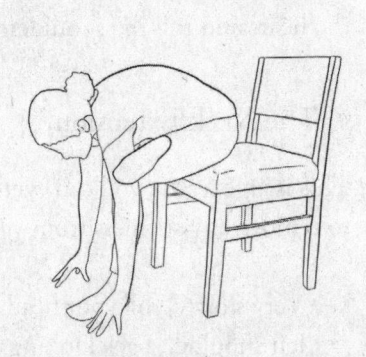

Step 1 of seated hip opener   Step 2 of seated hip opener

5

BRAIN-BOOSTING INFUSIONS

The easiest way to feel energized mid-afternoon (when cortisol levels dip) is with a cup of coffee. But while it may give you a shot of energy and alertness, for some (such as me), caffeine can be so stimulating that it can lead to palpitations. Given that caffeine takes about 8 hours to metabolize, your afternoon cuppa could be the reason you're sleepless at night.

There are several herbal decoctions that are low on caffeine but enhance cognitive function and calm the mind. Tulsi and gotu kola are my favourites to calm the mind. I've written about both in my previous book. But nature has many more remedies beyond these potent herbs to enhance focus, boost memory and de-stress the mind.

✿ Brahmi

Brahmi is used as a generic name for two different herbs: *centella asiatica* and *bacopa monnieri*. The former is gotu kola, but the one I'm talking about is the latter. Gotu kola can be

identified by its large, circular leaves, whereas brahmi grows in wetlands and has small leaves with tiny white flowers. Both herbs work beautifully for the brain; but while gotu kola is more calming, brahmi works specifically to enhance memory. The other difference is that gotu kola is used in skincare for its ability to heal wounds, whereas brahmi is used often in haircare for its ability to boost brain function.

Brahmi works as an antioxidant and adaptogen as it helps the mind cope with added stress. Several studies prove that bacopa is a valuable herb that increases memory retention, prevents cognitive decline, preserves cellular health of brain tissues, and may reduce the risk of neuro-generative disorders and diseases. A lot of the tea labelled as brahmi is actually centella asiatica, so please check the ingredients to get authentic bacopa monnieri.

Take 1 teaspoon of dried brahmi leaf, pour freshly boiled water over it. Let steep for 5 minutes and drink up.

✪ Mulethi

Yashti madhu, liquorice or *mulethi*—all names for a herb that has multi-pronged benefits for the skin, body and brain. Used as a mask to clear pigmentation, its extract is also effective for some of those who are suffering from eczema and dermatitis. Its usage for throat infections and indigestion is well-documented in traditional medicine. However, not many people know that it may also work as a memory enhancer. Especially during times of stress, mulethi works to calm the mind and enhance learning, therefore, it's no surprise that it helps students during examinations.

Mulethi falls under the category of *medhya* or brain herbs in Ayurveda. The roots of this plant are being studied to understand its potential as an anti-depressant, anti-inflammatory and its brain protective properties. Keep in mind that this herb is mildly oestrogenic and can be toxic in high, continued doses. A high dose means anything above 10 grams every day, i.e. 2 teaspoons, which is impossible to consume. Take a break from this herb after three months of usage.

Use mulethi root especially during changing seasons, when we're prone to coughs and infections. Add a small, 1 inch of root (or half teaspoon mulethi powder) to your cup of chai, or boil it along with cardamom, tulsi, saffron and ginger to make a warming winter decoction. Let cool a bit, stir in a spoonful of raw honey and drink.

✿ Mint Leaves

All types of mint works well as a digestifs. Both spearmint and peppermint teas have been found to have benefits such as reduced bloating, pain, heartburn and acid reflux. Spearmint in particular is known to help reduce levels of testosterone in cases of PCOD and PCOS. Two cups of tea a day is believed to inhibit mild hirsutism and hormone-related acne related to these conditions. Research has also shown that spearmint extract helps improve memory in older adults, and also helps reduce stress by easing the mind. Peppermint is mostly used for its digestive benefits and also helps refresh the palate. Anecdotal evidence shows that it also helps refresh the mind by relieving headaches.

Brew the tea by pouring freshly boiled water over leaves. Let steep for at least 5 minutes before drinking.

✿ Teas

There's a reason why a cup of tea always makes you feel good, whether it is black, white or green. The active ingredient in tea is L-theanine, which promotes relaxation without making you drowsy. As it elevates levels of feel-good chemicals such as GABA, serotonin and dopamine, it also reduces chemicals that increase stress. In addition to these benefits, this compound modulates the alpha state in the mind, which is prevalent when you're relaxed or meditating. It also improves sleep, increases focus, reduces anxiety and helps maintain a healthy weight (obviously, if the other aspects of diet and exercise are in place).

Tea is the most common source of L-theanine, with black tea containing the maximum amount. However, since black tea also contains the highest dose of caffeine, it is prudent to keep it limited to no more than two cups a day. In the last decade, green tea has also surged in popularity. It is supremely popular for its antioxidant benefits, and many enjoy the astringent flavour of green tea around the world. While it deservedly leads the way among other herbal teas for its catechin called epigallocatechin-3-gallate (EGCG), most people aren't aware of its anxiety-fighting benefits. It has been found that green tea helps improve sleep and reduce stress. Animal studies on matcha (powdered green tea) have also reflected its anxiety-fighting potential. Ditto for black and white tea.

But the preparation of white and green teas must be done with care. While you can brew black tea with boiling water, white, green and matcha are prepared best with slighter cooler temperatures to preserve the active nutrients. White and green are best at 80 degree Celsius, while matcha works well with a lower temperature of 70-75 degree Celsius.

☼ Aparajita

This common backyard creeper has a multitude of benefits. It is utilized in the treatment of diabetes in traditional medicine and is considered to be a boon for beauty-related concerns. Believed to increase the thickness of hair and halt premature ageing of the skin, the flowers are also used to make a bright blue tea which helps calm the mind and increase focus. Very little scientific literature is available for these benefits; however, it is cited several times in ayurvedic classics such as *Charaka Samhita*, *Sushruta Samhita* and *Ashtanga Hridayam*. In these classics, it is mentioned as a valuable memory enhancer, which has the ability to eliminate mental exhaustion. It is also believed to help enhance intelligence, refine the voice and improve digestion.

However, just like there are two brahmis in Ayurveda, there is confusion between *aparajita* and *shankhapushpi*, as both are shaped like a conch shell, its ayurvedic description. Both plants come under the medhya or brain-enhancing category in Ayurveda. Even though shankhapushpi is identified as a different flower in north India, in the south, both are considered to have similar powers.

To brew the tea, pour freshly boiled water over aparajita flowers and let steep till the water turns a deep blue colour. If you add a few drops of lemon juice, the colour changes to light pink. If you want some sweetness, add a bit of honey. You can also make this as an iced tea in summer.

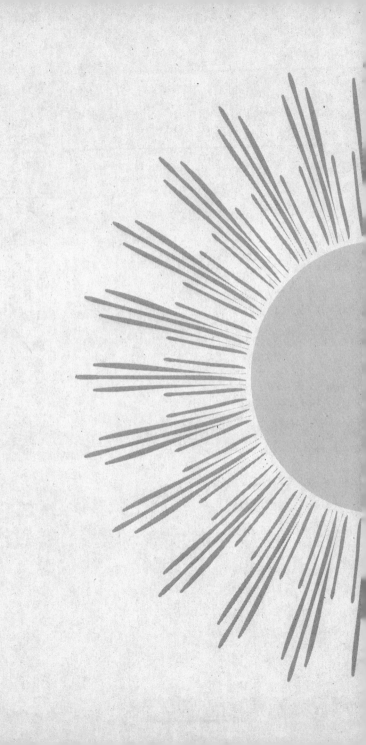

PILLAR III

✳

Focus

When you find the Buddha, kill him.

—Japanese koan

I first learnt about Japanese koans at a Zen retreat in southern Japan. Written as phrases or short stories, koans refine the mind via contemplation. Zen monks focus on them for hours, days or months, until one day, after the debris of the mind is swept away, the answer becomes crystal clear. This koan in particular refers to our need to look outside of ourselves for relief. It says destroy any external source of salvation (Buddha), because you already contain everything you need. Of course, there are many interpretations of this koan. If you look at it another day, it could mean something entirely different. But for me, it means to sweep away expectations, so that realizations come forth with clarity.

Contemplation helps refine the mind as long as we can observe the flow of our thoughts, which requires immense focus. It's natural to become a participant in the thought process, which makes too involved in our stories, making the mind scattered as it jumps from one assumption to another. This is why focus—defined by one-pointedness or convergence of attention—requires immense mental stamina. While achieving it may be easy, sustaining it requires practice.

So just like we exercise our muscles regularly to maintain strength and flexibility, the mind also requires regular practice to increase powers of concentration.

Meditation is nothing but an exercise for the mind. Though many think that just sitting down to meditate magically erases all thoughts, the reality is quite far from this assumption. It's impossible not to think, but after years of practice, the thoughts become fewer. At a vipassana retreat, I learnt that the trick to meditation is to treat the mind like a child. Every time it runs away, bring it back to the practice, again and again, without getting agitated. With practice, one becomes aware when thoughts travel so that we can choose to bring it back to the point of focus.

Though we live in a world that values multitasking, to refine the mind, we need repetition of the same task so it gets habituated to focus. Research proves that multitasking adds immense mental stress and creates negativity. What's more, people are more productive when they focus on one task at a time. Our brains are hardwired to go in and out of focus. At an average, the human mind brings its attention out of a task and surveys the surroundings. It's an adaptive technique that harks back to a time when humans had to scan the surroundings for perceived threats such as predators. For a mind that is already distracted, working on several things at a time means that the brain does not become sharper but more scattered.

To mine a precious resource, we need to tap away at one point till we strike gold. Meditative practices that polish the intellect are usually repetitive and one-pointed. Today spiritual shopping is the newest lifestyle trend. It provides

a fertile ground to delve into and experiment with several practices. It's a great way to find what works for you, but then one must stick to that one method. I must confess that I too have indulged in several spiritual practices. But as I solidify my rituals, I understand the profound effects of adhering regularly to one style.

There is no doubt that the brain must be challenged with new activities. Whether it's learning a new language or solving puzzles, any newness creates fresh neural pathways in the brain to make it quicker and more intelligent. Therefore, rituals help add a newness that keeps the mind fresh and practiced for focus. But though new activity helps exercise the mind, sharpening focus requires a single activity that can gather scattered thoughts and condense them into a line of thought. It doesn't have to take hours, even a short 5-10 minutes, consistent practice will do. Short spells of repetitive activity not only gets you habituated to concentration, but also used to boredom, the enemy of focus. It doesn't just have to be pranayama of meditation. The practice of *trataka* or candle meditation helps enhance concentration, as you centre you attention on the flame of a candle or diya.

Of course, many practices can and do work beautifully together. However, in this day and age, where free time is precious and guidance rare, it is prudent to choose one technique and stick to it. There may be times that a practice may not suit you. I've tried many different techniques and found that there were several that depleted my energies instead of multiplying them. Then there were other methods that made me feel anxious. The right practice for you should

(over a period of time) make you feel grounded, centred, calm, focus and energized.

In this section, you'll find many tools for centring the mind. There are balancing poses, mudras, mantras and mindfulness that can be woven harmoniously with simple meditations. While this is a great toolkit to enhance focus and concentration, it does not replace a meditation school or training under the tutelage of an experienced teacher. Guided meditations are convenient, but to advance in your daily practices, there is no replacement of learning from an experienced teacher.

I love the concept of the beginners mind, from Master Shunryu Suzuki book *Zen Mind, Beginner's Mind*. Though it seems like a tall order, but practicing with a fresh mind is key to finding satisfaction in repetitive tasks. It's like reading the Gita over and over again, or meditating with the same technique year after year. The method or content may remain the same but there is always a new discovery, a eureka moment, of unearthing something new about yourself. As Suzuki writes, 'If your mind is empty, it is always ready for anything; it is open to everything. In the beginner's mind there are many possibilities; in the expert's mind there are few.'

1

TRATAKA

Many successful people are habitual procrastinators as it is human nature to remain in the comfort zone. It's comforting for the mind to jump from one thought to another, whereas focusing on a single activity is hard work. Ultimately, the brain is an extension of the body and must be given the same attention. Therefore, just like we train and develop bodily functions with exercise, the mind too can be developed with certain practices done with consistency.

I noticed the changes in my mind after I spent ten days at a vipassana retreat, with 10 hours of daily meditation. It was a brain bootcamp, where I learnt to sharpen my mind and developed the habit of not jumping from one thought to another. I didn't notice the change until I came back to work. Before the retreat, it would take me some time to get down to work. After vipassana, I'd begin straightaway and write without procrastination. Of course, an intensive retreat like this may not suit everyone. However, there are many things you can do to develop focus.

Cultivating Internal Vision

Trataka is an ancient yogic practice to increase concentration and improve eye health. Some limit its definition to candle meditation, but this practice goes beyond just staring at a flame. You can focus at a *bindu* on a wall, the image of your deity, the aum sign, the full moon or the rising and setting sun. The flame of a candle is the most common tool for practising trataka, because there's something about its several layers that make it very mesmerizing and easy to focus upon. Because it has several layers, colours, transparency and opaqueness, it's an interesting, engaging visual.

Though this practice helps increase focus, but being one of the *shat kriyas* (the six cleansing techniques), it also helps purify the eyes. As the tears flow during this practice, they take with them the impurities from the socket. The eyes are the seat of pitta or fire, it is believed traditionally that staring at a form of fire helps the eye regain its functions, including eyesight. Small studies have shown that this practice along with eye exercises definitely holds the potential to improve sight.

Personally, I like it because it feels like a deep cleanse for the eyes. Even though we scrupulously wash every part of our body and clear our mind with several practices, the eyes get no special cleansing, despite being the most utilized organ in the modern world—we're constantly staring at our phones and laptops without providing the eyes any relief. There's a reason why crying feels detoxifying, because tears take away the film of build-up, washing and renewing the eyes from within. This is what trataka does, a deep cleanse without the heartbreak.

In terms of focus, I've certainly found my attention to be better during meditation when I practice trataka beforehand, even if it's only for a couple of minutes. While there is no doubt that this holds potential in improving focus and concentration over the long term, there is an immediate improvement as well. Studies have also found immediate cognitive benefits following trataka, be it better attention or problem-solving abilities. However, as it is with all traditional practices, there isn't any definite proof of improvement. The only benefits are experienced and anecdotal.

The ancient yogic text, *The Hatha Yoga Pradipika*, claims that trataka erases all diseases associated with vision. Because we also consume through our eyes, it is believed that staring at a single object and gazing at it internally develops your intuition. The word for single-pointed focus is *ekagrata*. This is the perfect word to summarize the practice: steady gaze, steady mind, steady life.

To do:

1) Sit in a darkened room—if there is any source of light it must come from behind, not in front of you.
2) Place a candle at eye level, at an arm's distance from you. Make sure there isn't any draft in the room, because the flame needs to be steady and not flickering.
3) If you can light a diya instead of a candle, that would be ideal. You can use either ghee, sesame or castor oil; castor oil being the most preferred since it produces the brightest flame.

4) Stare at the candle flame till your eyes tear up. Do not blink and do not keep shifting your gaze. Only close your eyes when they're filled with tears.

5) Then close your eyes, but do not rub them. Open again and stare at the flame.

6) You can begin by practising this for 2 minutes and then close your eyes. You will see an image of the flame in your mind's eye. If it moves, try to bring that flame to the point between your brows, also known as the *ajna chakra* or the third eye.

7) Once the image disappears, open your eyes and stare at the flame again.

8) Practise this meditation starting with 5 and going up to 20 minutes.

9) If you are epileptic, do not practise the candle trataka. Consult a yoga teacher about the best meditation for you.

10) Do not focus too hard, don't harden your eyes, keep your eyes and mind, both soft and receptive.

Tip: Never wear eye cream or sunscreen while doing trataka as these products can get into the eyes and cause stinging.

2

EYE EXERCISES

Though our eyes have a wide range of movement, being able to rotate in several different directions, we tend to utilize them to mostly look straight or sideways. Technology has compounded this static stare at our phones and computers with a few blinks for respite. But just like we need move our spine in all different directions in yoga to keep it flexible, eyes need exercise too. Practised regularly, these simple steps not only relax and refresh the eyes but also build strength.

Palming

Constant squinting and straining stresses the eyes and to a certain degree, how we use them determines their health. Palming is one of the most comforting exercises as it relaxes the optical nerve. While it is better to do palming in a darkened room to harness its complete range of benefits, practise it when you need a break from work. All you need to do is rub your palms together till they're warm and then place

them on the eyes. Keep them on the lids so that the warmth can permeate deep within. Remove and rub palms together for a second round while keeping your eyes closed. Practice 3-5 rounds.

Blinking

Sometimes we have dry eyes because we're so engrossed in work that we just forget to blink. This exercise is fairly simple—just blink the eyes quickly 10-12 times and then close your eyes for a few breaths. Open again and repeat. Do 3-5 rounds of this technique. This helps reduce dry eye.

Sideways

Stretch your arms out towards the sides, fists closed and thumbs up. Shift the arms slightly ahead of the shoulders so you can see the thumbs when you move the eyes to the side. Then without moving the neck, roll the pupil towards the right, bring the gaze back to the centre and then towards the left. Practice about 10 rounds each—one round includes gazing both towards the left and right thumb.

Circular

Close one eye with one palm and extend the other palm out in front of you. fist closed, thumb up. Now rotate the arm in a large circle, keeping the eyes fixed on the thumb. Rotate the arm 10 times each, both clockwise and anticlockwise.

Near and Distant

This can be practised by focusing on your thumbs—one kept close to the nose and the other extended away from you. You can also focus on an object close to you and then focus on something far away in the distance. Repeat 10 times.

Benefits

Even though there is some anecdotal evidence, which claims these exercises help with sight, there isn't any conclusive evidence or studies to prove that they can reverse changes. Still, there's no doubt that eye strain is a reality in the modern age. Eye exercises reduce the strain on the eyes by moving them in different directions. Think about it—if we keep sitting in one position all day, there is bound to be pain in the part that is bearing the weight. The same goes for our eyes. Therefore, moving them around helps reduce stress and increase focus.

If practising eye exercises doesn't fit into your schedule, try the 20-20-20 rule. While working on your computer, take a break every 20 minutes to look at something about 20 feet away, for 20 seconds.

3

BALANCING POSES

Yoga is primarily viewed as an exercise for the naturally flexible, which of course can discourage the inflexible ones to give it a try. But my favourite poses in yoga are not the ones that increase flexibility, but those that improve balance. Whether it's standing on one leg, on your toes or lifting up on your arms, these poses clearly reflect the state of your mind. With time, the practice of balances centres a scattered brain and refines powers of concentration. Of course, you could make your practice intensive with advanced balancing poses, but keeping it as simple as just balancing on leg will enhance your focus.

We know now that physical and mental health is interconnected. When you build physical endurance, mental stamina increases as a by-product. Similarly, when you improve balance in the body, it mirrors in the mind. Because developing focus is a matter of habit, whether you do it via meditation or physical practices. By adding a bit of balance in your daily routine, you can train your mind to focus.

There are three things that must be kept in mind while practising balance:

✿ Forgive your imbalance

When it comes to any form of exercise, our egos are intertwined with performance. This expectation of a superhuman performance without prior experience usually comes in the way of us sticking to a fitness routine. Drop the expectation and accept the imbalance. This is the first step.

✿ Fix your gaze

If you keep shifting your gaze in several directions, you will be unsteady. Keep your gaze stable, fixed at a point either in front of you or a few paces ahead on the floor. For beginners, keeping the gaze steady at the floor provides better balance.

✿ Soften your gaze

You needn't harden your gaze, in order to concentrate at a point. Be gentle with your focus to make it a habit. Soft eyes equal soft mind, and vice versa. I learnt this from two Iyengar teachers and it improved my yoga practice, making it much more enjoyable.

You can practice either one or all three poses 3-4 times a week:

The Tree Pose

This is a weight-bearing asana and is therefore excellent to improve bone health provided it's done correctly. It's easy

and simple to practise can be done every day to enhance your powers of concentration:

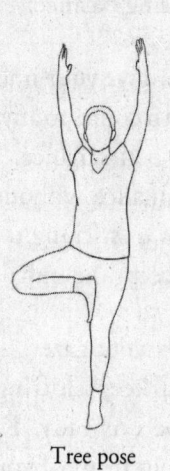

Tree pose

- ✪ Stand up tall and align your spine: knees aligned with the ankles, hips in the same line as the knees, pelvis neither too forward or back, chest (open with the shoulders pulled back) aligned over the pelvis.
- ✪ Rotate your right toes towards the right, then lift them up and place them either on the calf or near the groin. Do not place them on the knee as it will put unnecessary pressure on the joints.
- ✪ You can keep your palms in namaste position or lift them up.
- ✪ Keep your gaze fixed at a point.
- ✪ Begin by holding it for 5 breaths, work it up to 25 deep breaths on each leg.
- ✪ Repeat on the other leg.
- ✪ If you have problems with balance then you can also take support of the wall in the beginning.

Mountain Pose

When I was teaching, this pose would come at the beginning of my class. Not only does it help in balance, but it also strengthens the legs.

- ☼ Stand straight, imagining a centre line running through your body. Keep the knees over ankles, pelvis over hips, chest open without arching the back too much.
- ☼ Inhale and lift high on your toes (it helps if you do this barefoot with toes spread wide). Lift your arms up, keep them parallel to each other as you inhale.

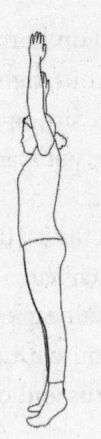

Mountain pose

- ☼ Hold for 5-10 breaths, come down on an exhale bringing your arms down with you.
- ☼ Repeat 3-5 times.

The Simple Eagle Pose

This pose is a little complicated, but is my absolute favourite because it instantly reflects the state of your mind. The day you're calm, you'll find the pose easy, but the days you're scattered, so the pose will be unsteady. While this is true for all balancing asanas, it is more relevant for this pose. The eagle eye is all about perfect concentration, therefore this is essential to sharpen your mind.

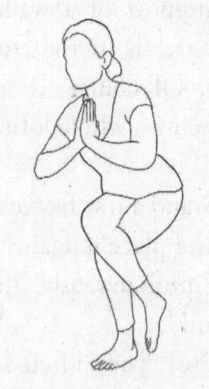

Simple eagle pose

- Stand on both feet and then squat.
- Lift your right leg and take it over your left knee, like you're sitting cross-legged on a chair.
- Bring your arms in namaste position in front of your chest.
- Hold for 5-10 breaths and change your leg. Do three reps on each leg.
- The full eagle pose is when you loop the foot around the calf muscle and interlace both arms but, for the purpose of focus and concentration, just this variation is enough.

Supported Dancers Pose

The reason this asana is so loved is because it's a backbend and balancing pose in one. But instead of doing the traditional *nataraj* asana, I like to take the support of a walk to get a nice stretch in the front of my body. Of course, it also makes balancing a whole lot easier.

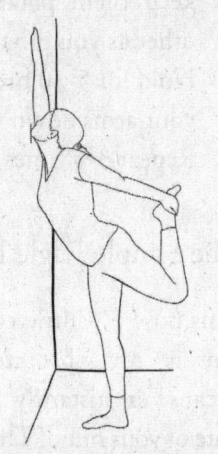

Supported dancer pose

- Stand a few feet away from a wall. Lift your right arm up and place it against the wall.
- Simultaneously lift your left leg and grab hold of the ankle.
- Push your lifted foot back into the palm so that your entire body arches forward.

- ✿ You should feel a stretch in your right armpit, waist, hip flexor and thigh.
- ✿ Hold the pose for a minimum 10 breaths or a bit longer as it is supported variation.
- ✿ Repeat on the other side and practice 3 reps.

4

MUDRA

The science of mudra teaches is that everything good is available to us right at our fingertips. Though this practice is seen mostly as hand gestures, mudras also include several body positions, including the more relaxed shoulder stand, also known as the *viprita karni*. The literal meaning and purpose of mudra is the same—to work as a seal, to prevent loss of prana, life force, qi or energy.

To understand how it works, put a 1-minute timer on your phone, close your eyes and observe your thoughts. Now do it again with your hands in the chin the mudra, where the tips of the thumb and forefinger touch each other. Remember that the contact between the fingers has to be nail-to-nail so the nerve-endings at the end of your fingertips come into contact. If you observe carefully, you'll find that while your thoughts seem more scattered when your hands are not in a gesture, with the mudra, the mind feels slightly more contained.

If you focus on the sensation in your fingertips touching each other, you will also feel a vibration. This isn't to say

that meditation is only possible with a hand gesture, but it certainly helps seal the prana or contain the mind. In a small experiment a group of practitioners were studied practising the prana mudra. Electrophotonic imaging (EPI) captured the coronal discharge—electrical release surrounding a conductor that carries high voltage—around the fingers. Though there wasn't much change in EPI imaging with 5 minutes of mudra practice, there were significant changes in the imagery by day three with a 20-minute mudra practice. Even though this isn't very conclusive, this does show that mudra is in fact a science, which can be utilized for energy manipulation.

I first experienced the blissful effect of mudra practice after I was taught the yoni mudra by an ayurvedic doctor in Pune. This mudra is supposed to be beneficial for gynaecological problems, but I didn't practise it with regularity for it to benefit me physically. Still, I felt the mental effects immediately. The doctor who taught me the mudra told me it would give me a feeling of protection and safety, which it did. Even today, every time I feel restless or scattered, I practice the yoni mudra to make me feel calm and centred again.

Mudra and the Five Elements

Mudras are an ancient practice, some believe even older than yoga. In fact, mudra isn't yogic, even though it is now used to complement pranayama and meditation. It is originally part of tantra, where *bandhas* (locks) and mudras were considered to do the same thing, i.e., work with energy and seal it within the body. If you've practised yoga, you know the simplest

bandhas are the ones in which you either pull in your stomach or tuck in your chin to create a sort of seal to prevent loss of prana, which is also considered to be a mudra. But in this chapter, I will primarily talk about hand gestures.

In Ayurveda or TCM, it is believed that we are made of the five elements: fire, water, earth, air and space. Each finger corresponds to each of these elements. The thumb is for fire, forefinger is air, middle is space, ring finger for earth, and the little finger for water. When you touch the tip of the thumb to any other fingertip, it amplifies that particular element. And if you use the thumb to press down a finger, it will reduce that element. Of course, these are just the basics. The mudra science is vast and complicated. Many believe that several ailments can be healed just with the right mudras. While there isn't any scientific evidence to support this claim, I can say from personal experience that adding hand gestures to your daily regimen is a great method to centre the mind and enhance meditative practices, and perhaps even boost physical health. Like any meditative ritual, start by practicing this for short periods between 2-5 minutes and slowly build it up to 15-30 minutes.

Enhance awareness with . . .

Chinmaya Mudra

Though the most popular mudra to create peace of mind and awareness is the gyan mudra, I find something very comforting in the closed fists of the *chinmaya mudra*. This gesture is used to calm the nerves and enhance awareness, and some claim

that it even helps in weight loss. I assume it's because the thumb (fire) meets with the forefinger (air), and the heavier elements of space (middle finger), earth (ring finger) and water (little finger) are turned inwards. Of course, diet and exercise would also need to go along with a mudra to facilitate weight loss, but its uses and finger placement are

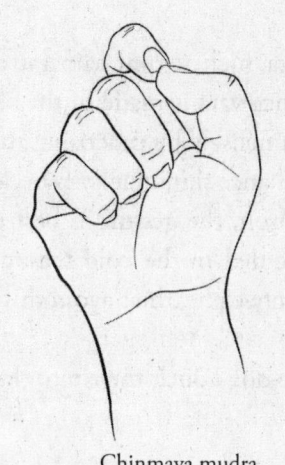

Chinmaya mudra

fascinating. The gesture also helps improve the flow of energy and memory and reduces anxiety.

To do: Curl the fingers of the palm into a fist. Touch the tips of the thumb and forefinger so they form a circle. Place hand on the upper thighs, either facing upwards or downwards as per your comfort.

Improve skin with . . .

Varun Mudra

The *varun mudra* is said to increase hydration in the body as the little finger stands for the water element. Because it helps with fluid balance, it also helps improve circulation and reduce ailments that are caused by high

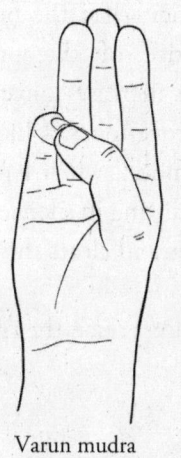

Varun mudra

vata, such as joint pain and also pitta problems such as acidity. Since vata is made of the air and space elements, it is helped immensely by practising this mudra. The reason it is said to enhance skin quality is because it increases moisture. For this reason, the gesture is best practised in summer months and avoided in the cold season. If you have cough, cold or are overweight, then avoid this mudra.

To do: Touch the tip of the little finger and the thumb.

Energize yourself with . . .

Prana Mudra

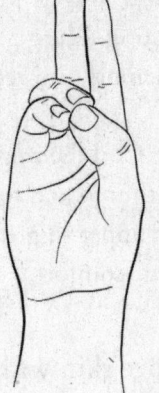

This was the mudra practised in the small study mentioned earlier in this chapter. With a combination of fire, earth and water, this mudra is extremely balancing for the body. Regular practice of the prana gesture helps increase concentration and

Prana mudra

improve focus. I like to practise this mudra around the late afternoon, when I need to work but don't have the energy. Just sitting in silence with my fingers pressed into this gesture calms and clears the mind by removing fatigue.

To do: Touch the tips of the thumb, ring and little finger.

Improve digestion with . . .

Apana Mudra

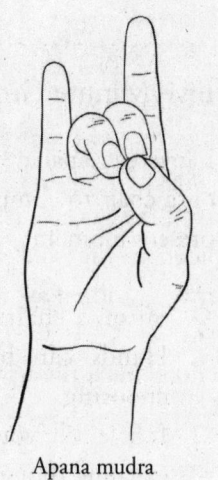

If prana is the energy flow that goes in the upwards direction, apana is the opposite and flows downward. Prana and apana are also two of the five vayus or energy channels in the body. Prana rules the lungs and chest, while apana rules the lower organs of

Apana mudra

digestion, reproduction and elimination. Therefore, the apana gesture isn't just beneficial for digestion but also menstruation. In Ayurveda, it is believed that most gynaecological problems are caused by a blocked apana vayu, which basically means that the downward flow of energy is restricted.

To do: Touch the tips of your thumb, ring and middle fingers. Focus on the sensation between the fingers or the downward flow of energy. Practice every day for 15-30 minutes.

Five-Minute Grounding Practice

I love the apana vayu breathing practice while sitting on a chair to eliminate stress and ground myself in the present moment:

- ✿ Sit on a chair with both feet flat on the ground. Hands can be loose or in a mudra of your choosing.
- ✿ Inhale till your pelvis, and then imagine you're exhaling though your feet. Repeat 10 or 25 times.
- ✿ You can also do this in the garden with bare feet on the grass.

Ground yourself with . . .

Yoni Mudra

If you want a break from the constant chatter in the mind, the yoni mudra gives you the feeling of protection and calmness, sort of like in your mother's womb. All the fingers in this pose are interlaced and pressed together, therefore

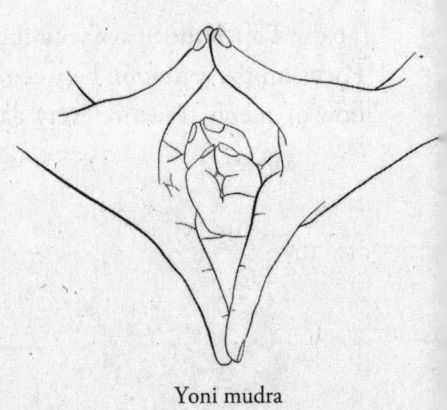

Yoni mudra

it helps balance the left and right hemispheres of the brain. Needless to say, this gesture is excellent for reproductive

health and can be practised alongside mainstream medicine if you have PCOS or endometriosis. But if you need a break and just want to retreat into the stillness of your mind, this mudra is ideal.

To do: Place the back of the palms against each other. Then interlace the middle, ring and little fingers so that the tips of the left and right fingers are pressing against each other from the inside of your palms. Extend the forefingers downwards and thumbs upwards with the tips pressed together. It should look like a yoni shape. Place it in front of your pelvis and hold for 15 minutes or upwards.

BIBLIOGRAPHY

Introduction

'Sun Fact Sheet.' https://nssdc.gsfc.nasa.gov/planetary/factsheet/sunfact.html.

American Heart Association News. 'Could sunshine lower blood pressure? Study offers enlightenment'. 28 February 2020. https://www.heart.org/en/news/2020/02/28/could-sunshine-lower-blood-pressure-study-offers-enlightenment.

Facer-Childs, E. R., Middleton, B., Skene, D. J., and Bagshaw, A. P. 'Resetting the late timing of "night owls" has a positive impact on mental health and performance.' *Sleep medicine*. 60, (2019): 236–247. https://doi.org/10.1016/j.sleep.2019.05.001.

Farhud D, Aryan Z. 'Circadian Rhythm, Lifestyle and Health: A Narrative Review.' *Iran J Public Health*. 47(8) (August 2018):1068-1076. https://www.ncbi.nlm.nih.gov/pmc/articles/PMC6123576/.

Fisk, Angus S., Tam, Shu K. E., Brown, Laurence A., Vyazovskiy, Vladyslav V., Bannermant, David M. and Peirson, Stuart N. 'Light and Cognition: Roles for Circadian Rhythms, Sleep, and Arousal'. *Frontiers in Neurology*. 9 (2018). https://www.frontiersin.org/articles/10.3389/fneur.2018.00056.

Kasof, Joseph. 'Indoor lighting preferences and bulimic behavior: An individual differences approach.' *Personality and Individual*

Differences—PERS INDIV DIFFER. 32 (2002): 383-400. https://www.researchgate.net/publication/247167126_Indoor_lighting_preferences_and_bulimic_behavior_An_individual_differences_approach.

Mead M.N. 'Benefits of sunlight: a bright spot for human health.' *Environ Health Perspect.* 116(4) (2008):A160-A167. doi:10.1289/ehp.116-a160.

Nemo, Leslie. 'Spending Time in the Sun Might Make Your Gut Healthier'. *Discover.* (25 October 2019). https://www.discovermagazine.com/health/spending-time-in-the-sun-might-make-your-gut-healthier.

Ondrusova, K., Fatehi, M., Barr, A., et al. 'Subcutaneous white adipocytes express a light sensitive signaling pathway mediated via a melanopsin/TRPC channel axis.' *Sci Rep* 7, 16332 (2017). https://doi.org/10.1038/s41598-017-16689-4.

Randler, Christoph. 'Defend Your Research: The Early Bird Really Does Get the Worm'. *Harvard Business Review.* (July-August 2010). https://hbr.org/2010/07/defend-your-research-the-early-bird-really-does-get-the-worm.

Purify

'Multitasking: Switching costs'. *American Psychological Association.* https://www.apa.org/topics/research/multitasking.

'Washing the hands makes us feel more optimistic – study'. *European Cleaning Journal* (25 November 2013). http://www.europeancleaningjournal.com/magazine/articles/latest-news/washing-the-hands-makes-us-feel-more-optimistic-study.

AMLA—Grover HS, et al. 'Therapeutic effects of amla in medicine and dentistry: A review'. *J Oral Res Rev* [serial online].7 (2015): 65-8. https://www.jorr.org/text.asp?2015/7/2/65/172498.

ANANTAMOOL— Chakrabortty, Sumona and Choudhary, Rachana. 'HEMIDESMUS INDICUS (ANANTMOOL): RARE HERB OF CHHATTISGARH'. *Indian J.Sci.Res.*4 (1) (2014): 89-93. https://www.ijsr.in/upload/1551655300.

BATHS—Rao, B. Rama. 'Bath in Ayurveda, Yoga and Dharmasastra'. http://www.ccras.nic.in/sites/default/files/viewpdf/jimh/BIIHM_1982/13%20to%2021.pdf.

BEETS—Mirmiran, P., et al. 'Functional properties of beetroot (*Beta vulgaris*) in management of cardio-metabolic diseases'. *Nutr Metab* (Lond) 17:3 (7 January 2020). doi: 10.1186/s12986-019-0421-0.

BEETS—Petrie, M., et al. 'Beet Root Juice: An Ergogenic Aid for Exercise and the Aging Brain'. *J Gerontol A Biol Sci Med Sci.* 72(9) (1 September 2017):1284-1289. doi: 10.1093/gerona/glw219.

CHIA SEED—Roizen, Michael F. and Oz, Mehmet. *You: Staying Young: The Owner's Manual for Extending your Warranty.* (New York: Scribner, 2007).

CHIA SEED—Ullah R, Nadeem M, et al. 'Nutritional and therapeutic perspectives of Chia (Salvia hispanica L.): a review'. *Food Sci Technol.* 53(4) (April 2016):1750-8. doi: 10.1007/s13197-015-1967-0.

COPPER WATER—Sudha VB, Ganesan S, Pazhani GP, Ramamurthy T, Nair GB, Venkatasubramanian and P. 'Storing drinking-water in copper pots kills contaminating diarrhoeagenic bacteria'. *Health Popul Nutr.* 30(1) (March 2012):17-21. doi: 10.3329/jhpn.v30i1.11271.

CUMIN—Abdul-Jabar, Rafeef. 'Chemical analysis and antimicrobial activity of Cumin seeds extracted oil against some bacterial and fungal isolates'. *Thi-Qar Science.* 3. (2013): 65-73. https://www.researchgate.net/publication/318672358_Chemical_analysis_and_antimicrobial_activity_of_Cumin_

seeds_extracted_oil_against_some_bacterial_and_fungal_ isolates.

FASTING DETOX—Araveti, P.B., Srivastava, A. 'Curcumin induced oxidative stress causes autophagy and apoptosis in bovine leucocytes transformed by *Theileria annulata'. Cell Death Discov.* 5, 100 (2019). https://doi.org/10.1038/s41420-019-0180-8.

FASTING DETOX— 'Early Time-Restricted Feeding Improves Insulin Sensitivity, Blood Pressure, and Oxidative Stress Even without Weight Loss in Men with Prediabetes'. *Cell Metabolism.* Volume 27, Issue 6 (2018): 1212-1221.e3. https://doi.org/10.1016/j.cmet.2018.04.010.

FASTING DETOX—He, C, Sumpter, R Jr and Levine, B. 'Exercise induces autophagy in peripheral tissues and in the brain'. *Autophagy.* 8(10) (October 2018):1548-51. doi: 10.4161/auto.21327.

FASTING DETOX— Schiattarella GG and Hill JA. 'Therapeutic targeting of autophagy in cardiovascular disease'. *Mol Cell Cardiol.* 95(June 2016):86-93. doi: 10.1016/j.yjmcc.2015.11.019.

FASTING DETOX—Marinac CR, et al. 'Prolonged Nightly Fasting and Breast Cancer Prognosis'. *JAMA Oncol.* 2(8) (2016):1049–1055. doi:10.1001/jamaoncol.2016.0164.

FLAX SEED—Parikh, M, et al. 'Dietary Flaxseed as a Strategy for Improving Human Health'. *Nutrients.* 11(5) (25 May 2019):1171. doi: 10.3390/nu11051171.

HAIR CLEANSE—Banerjee, Pooja S., et al. 'Preparation, evaluation and hair growth stimulating activity of herbal hair oil'. *Journal of Chemical and Pharmaceutical Research* 1(1) (2009): 261-267. http://www.jocpr.com/articles/preparation-evaluation-and-hair-growth-stimulating-activity-of-herbal-hair-oil.pdf.

HERBS—Quispe, Cristina, et al. 'Chemical Composition and Antioxidant Activity of *Aloe vera* from the Pica Oasis (Tarapacá, Chile) by UHPLC-Q/Orbitrap/MS/MS'. *Journal of Chemistry*, vol. 2018 (2018). https://doi.org/10.1155/2018/6123850

HERBS—Maan, Abid, et al. 'The therapeutic properties and applications of Aloe vera : A review'. *Journal of Herbal Medicine*. (2018). 12. 10.1016/j.hermed.2018.01.002.

Hibiscus—Hopkins AL, et al. 'Hibiscus sabdariffa L. in the treatment of hypertension and hyperlipidemia: a comprehensive review of animal and human studies'. *Fitoterapia*. 85 (March 2013):84-94. doi: 10.1016/j.fitote.2013.01.003.

HONEY—Eteraf-Oskouei T, Najafi M. 'Traditional and modern uses of natural honey in human diseases: a review'. *Iran J Basic Med Sci*. 16(6)(June 2013):731-42. PMID: 23997898; PMCID: PMC3758027.

Kohara, K., Tabara, Y., Ochi, M., et al. 'Habitual hot water bathing protects cardiovascular function in middle-aged to elderly Japanese subjects.' *Sci Rep* 8, 8687 (2018). https://doi.org/10.1038/s41598-018-26908-1.

NETTLE—De Vico, Gionata, Guida, Vincenzo and Carella Francesca. 'Urtica dioica (Stinging Nettle): A Neglected Plant With Emerging Growth Promoter/Immunostimulant Properties for Farmed Fish'. *Frontiers in Physiology*. 9 (2018). https://www.frontiersin.org/articles/10.3389/fphys.2018.00285

NETTLE—Kar, Prasanna Kumar, Nath, Lilakanth, et al. 'Hepatoprotective Effect of the Ethanolic Extract of *Urtica parviflora* Roxb. in CCl4 Treated Rats.' *International Journal of Pharmacology*, 3 (2007): 362-366. https://scialert.net/fulltext/?doi=ijp.2007.362.366.

OIL PULLING—Shanbhag VK. 'Oil pulling for maintaining oral hygiene - A review'. *Tradit Complement Med*. 7(1)(6 June 2016):106-109. doi: 10.1016/j.jtcme.2016.05.004.

BIBLIOGRAPHY

ORAL HEALTH—Matsui, M., Chosa, N., Shimoyama, Y. *et al.* 'Effects of tongue cleaning on bacterial flora in tongue coating and dental plaque: a crossover study'. *BMC Oral Health* 14, 4 (2014). https://doi.org/10.1186/1472-6831-14-4.

ORAL HEALTH—Singh A, Purohit B. 'Tooth brushing, oil pulling and tissue regeneration: A review of holistic approaches to oral health'. *Ayurveda Integr Med.* 2(2) (April 2011):64-8. doi: 10.4103/0975-9476.82525.

R., Renjith. 'The Effect of Information Overload in Digital Media News Content'. (2017). https://www.researchgate. net/publication/324088772_The_Effect_of_Information_ Overload_in_Digital_Media_News_Content.

SABJA SEED—Munir, M., et al. 'Nutritional assessment of basil seed and its utilization in development of value added beverage'. *Pakistan Journal of Agricultural Research*, 30(3) (2017): 266-271.

Saxbe, D. E. and Repetti, R. 'No place like home: home tours correlate with daily patterns of mood and cortisol'. *Personality & social psychology bulletin*, *36*(1) (2010): 71–81. https://doi. org/10.1177/0146167209352864.

TONGUE SCRAPER—Pedrazzi, V., Sato, S., de Mattos, M., Lara, E. H., & Panzeri, H. 'Tongue-cleaning methods: a comparative clinical trial employing a toothbrush and a tongue scraper'. *Journal of periodontology 75*(7) (2004):1009–1012. https://doi.org/10.1902/jop.2004.75.7.1009.

TRIPHAL RINSE—Prakash S, Shelke AU. 'Role of Triphala in dentistry'. *Indian Soc Periodontol.* 18(2)(March 2014):132-5. doi: 10.4103/0972-124X.131299.

TRIPHALA EYE DROPS—Gangamma MP, Poonam, Rajagopala M. 'A clinical study on "Computer vision syndrome" and its management with Triphala eye drops and Saptamrita Lauha'. *Ayu.* 31(2)(April 2010):236-9. doi: 10.4103/0974-8520.72407.

VETIVER—Balasankar, D., et al. Traditional and medicinal uses of vetiver. *Med. Plants Stud.*. 1(2013): 191-200. https://www. researchgate.net/publication/285320583_Traditional_and_ medicinal_uses_of_vetiver.

WHEAT AND BARLEY GRASS—Qamar, Aiza, et al. 'Exploring the phytochemical profile of green grasses with special reference to antioxidant properties'. *International Journal of Food Properties*, 21:1 (2018): 2566-2577, DOI: 10.1080/10942912.2018.1540990.

WHEAT AND BARLEY GRASS—Zeng, Yawen, et al. 'Preventive and Therapeutic Role of Functional Ingredients of Barley Grass for Chronic Diseases in Human Beings'. *Oxidative Medicine and Cellular Longevity*, vol. 2018. https://doi. org/10.1155/2018/3232080.

WHEAT AND BARLEY GRASS—Deng R and Chow TJ. 'Hypolipidemic, antioxidant, and antiinflammatory activities of microalgae Spirulina'. *Cardiovasc Ther* (4) (28 August 2010): e33-45. doi: 10.1111/j.1755-5922.2010.00200.x.

WHEAT AND BARLEY GRASS—Gopalakrishnan, Lakshmipriya, et al. 'Moringa oleifera: A review on nutritive importance and its medicinal application'. *Food Science and Human Wellness*. Volume 5, Issue 2 (2016): 49-56. https://doi.org/10.1016/j. fshw.2016.04.001.

Energy

BREATH— Shankarappa V, et al. 'The Short Term Effect of Pranayama on the Lung Parameters'. (15 February 2012). https://www.jcdr.net/articles/PDF/1861/6%20-%203476. (A).pdf.

BREATH—Sharma VK, et al. 'Effect of fast and slow pranayama practice on cognitive functions in healthy volunteers'.

Clin Diagn Res. 8(1)(January 2014):10-3. doi: 10.7860/JCDR/2014/7256.3668. Epub 2013 Nov 18.

Yamanaka, Y, Motoshima, H and Uchida, K. 'Hypothalamic-pituitary-adrenal axis differentially responses to morning and evening psychological stress in healthy subjects'. *Neuropsychopharmacol Rep*. 39(2019): 41– 47. https://doi.org/10.1002/npr2.12042.

Focus

Gorlick, Adam. 'Media multitaskers pay mental price, Stanford study shows'. *Stanford Report*. (24 August 2009). https://news.stanford.edu/news/2009/august24/multitask-research-study-082409.html.

MORNING—Dolan, Eric W. 'Abstaining from smartphone use in the bedroom improves happiness, according to new research'. *PsyPost*. (11 April 2018). https://www.psypost.org/2018/04/abstaining-smartphone-use-bedroom-improves-happiness-according-new-research-51020.

MORNING—Elhai, J. D., et al. 'Problematic smartphone use: A conceptual overview and systematic review of relations with anxiety and depression psychopathology'. *Journal of affective disorders*, *207*(2017): 251–259. https://doi.org/10.1016/j.jad.2016.08.030.

MORNING—Matthay, M. A., et al. 'Acute respiratory distress syndrome'. *Nature reviews. Disease primers*. 5(1) (2019): 18. https://doi.org/10.1038/s41572-019-0069-0

MORNING—McFarlane SJ, et al. 'Alarm tones, music and their elements: Analysis of reported waking sounds to counteract sleep inertia'. *PLoS ONE* 15(1) (2020): e0215788. https://doi.org/10.1371/journal.pone.0215788.

MORNING—Peedikayil FC, et al. 'Effect of coconut oil in plaque related gingivitis - A preliminary report'. *Niger Med J.* 56(2) (March-April 2015):143-7. doi: 10.4103/0300-1652.153406.

MOVEMENT AND GESTURE—Howell, Nicholas A., et al. 'Association Between Neighborhood Walkability and Predicted 10-Year Cardiovascular Disease Risk: The CANHEART (Cardiovascular Health in Ambulatory Care Research Team) Cohort'. *Journal of the American Heart Association*. Vol.8, no. 21 (31 October 2019). https://www.ahajournals.org/doi/full/10.1161/JAHA.119.013146.

MOVEMENT AND GESTURE—Tigbe, W., Granat, M., Sattar, N. *et al.* Time spent in sedentary posture is associated with waist circumference and cardiovascular risk. *Int J Obes* 41, 689–696 (2017). https://doi.org/10.1038/ijo.2017.30.

MUDRA—Kumar KS, Srinivasan TM, Ilavarasu J, Mondal B and Nagendra HR. 'Classification of Electrophotonic Images of Yogic Practice of Mudra through Neural Networks'. *Int J Yoga*. 11(2) (May-August 2018):152-156. doi: 10.4103/ijoy. IJOY_76_16.

University of Houston. 'Multitasking in the workplace can lead to negative emotions: Study finds constant email interruptions create sadness and fear.' *ScienceDaily*. www.sciencedaily.com/releases/2020/05/200511154850.htm (accessed August 17, 2022).

Books for Sun

Flaws, Bob. *Curing Fibromyalgia Naturally With Chinese Medicine*. (Blue Poppy, 2000).

McBride, Shaman Melodie. *Going Towards the Nature Is Going Towards the Health*. (US: Xlibris, 2012).

Nishi, Katsuzo. *The Nishi System of Health Engineering*. (US: Kessinger Publishing, 2010).

Pitchford, Paul. *Healing with Whole Foods: Asian Traditions and Modern Nutrition*. (US: North Atlantic Books, 2002).

Saraswati, Swami Satyananda. *Asana Pranayama Mudra Bandha*. (Munger: Bihar School of Yoga, 2008).

Thompson, Richard L. *Vedic Cosmography and Astronomy*. (Motilal Banarsidass Publishers, 2003).

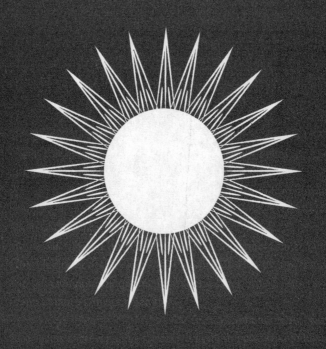

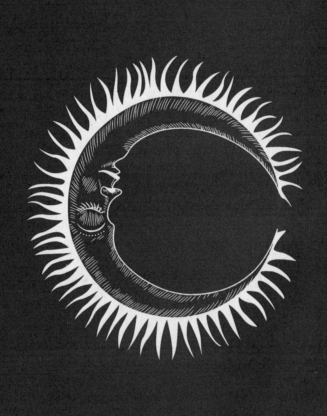